# Covid-19

# VISUALPERSPECTIVE

# ☆Flatten the Curve☆

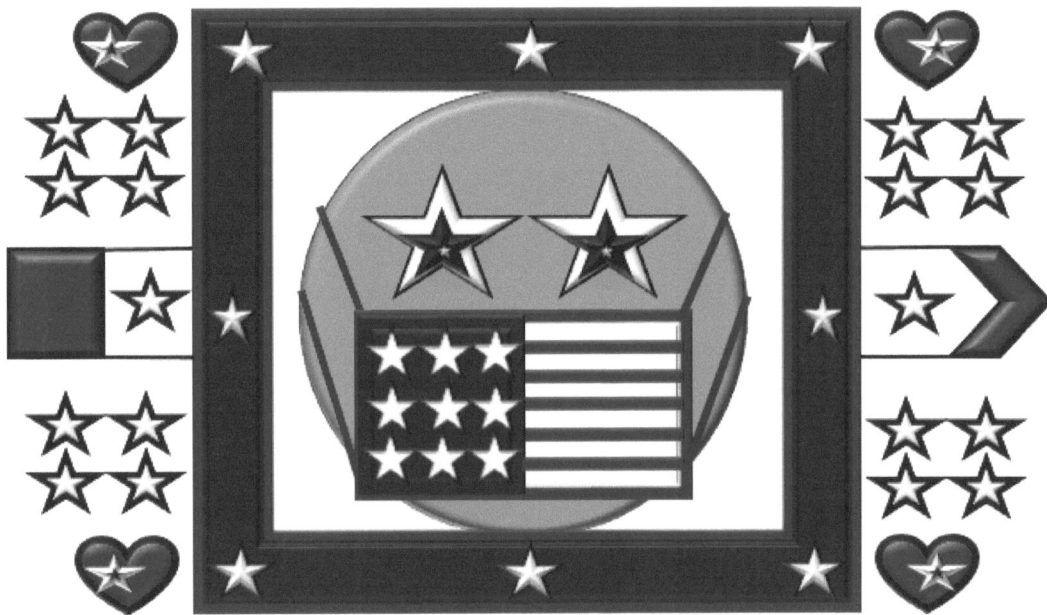

Exercises that Effectively Illustrate a Visual Perspective of the Impact SARS-CoV-2 novel coronavirus, Covid-19 is having in the United States.

My Personal Journey, Poetry, Thoughts, Facts on the Pandemic 2020.

Cheri Lemley, Resident of Washington State

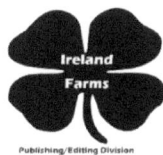

Editing and publishing consultant
Martha McKeeth Ireland
Ireland Farms Writer Services
Sequim, Washington

Ireland
Farms
Publishing/Editing Division

ISBN: 978-1-7356773-0-9

# Dedication

To the many, many families in mourning, my deepest condolences to you and yours. I pray for your comfort in this unfathomable time of grieving here in America and around the world.

To those on the Frontline, the doctors, nurses, EMTs and custodial staff who are providing essential care and sterilization at the risk of being unwittingly exposed to the Covid-19 virus.

You are literally the FRONTLINE!

You are America's heroes and heroines!

We appreciate you. Please know that many Americans do understand the seriousness of this pandemic. We truly are having a national emergency. I would like to believe everyone is taking every precaution humanly possible to avoid becoming infected with Covid-19. The numbers are telling a different story.

To the person who purchased this book(s) for themselves and or for others. Together we are saving lives!


Please take a moment, before proceeding, to watch the following **YouTube** video:

**ICU Nurse has a Powerful Message for Anti-Maskers | Now This**


Thank You,

With Compassion and Urgency,

A Covid-19 VisualPerspective,

Cheri Lemley 💜

# Contents

Please do your part to flatten the curve.

Why wear a mask?

There is so much controversy over the simple act of wearing a mask. Masks help prevent the spread of novel coronavirus and other infectious diseases. All N95 medical grade masks, reserved for the Frontline health care workers, are ideal for protecting people from the novel coronavirus. However, one of the biggest issues straight out the gate with this SARS-CoV-2 novel coronavirus #*%$#*@ pandemic is that there isn't/hasn't ever been enough N95 masks to even protect the Frontline Doctors and Nurses treating Covid19 patients! So we in the, "General Public" have been politely asked by the CDC, US Surgeon General, VADM Jerome M. Adams, M.D., M.P.H. to now wear whatever masks or face coverings we do have, to help prevent the spread of the novel coronavirus. Masks are an important part of our defense, as this **lethal virus** spreads person to person through respiratory droplets. Here in the NW one's breath is very visible on a cold wintery day. In the summertime (now) respiratory droplets, are usually as invisible as the virus, but they are nonetheless still there!  We have many more challenging days ahead of us.

An Invisible Enemy

<u>SARS-CoV-2 novel coronavirus</u>

WHO, World Health Organization

Names new virus on February 11, 2020


**S-** Severe

**A-** Acute

**R-** Respiratory

**S-** Syndrome –

**Co-** Corona

**V-** Virus

**2-** Genetically related to SARS (2003)


SARS-CoV-2 although related to SARS, is in fact new and different; hence, the term, "novel" coronavirus.

*"Numbers are interesting. We can make them say a lot of things. We can make them look like a lot of things, but behind those numbers are people. And you really don't want it to be you."*

Dr. Joseph Chang, chief medical officer of Parkland Hospital in Dallas, Texas in an interview referencing Covid-19, July 22, 2020

# Preface

So here I am, it is July and I am thinking back to January 1, 2020. It came in with a bang! "Not." In "hindsight," pun definitely intended; the Seattle Space Needle light show instead of fireworks, though cancelled due to high winds, should have been our first clue that something was amiss. For what it is worth, the Fire Department and those in charge actually acted very responsibly by putting on the alternative light show. And as much, we ourselves should be acting just as responsibly, now, in this historic moment in time by wearing our masks and or face coverings in public. We are in the middle of a World Pandemic for crying out loud! A National Emergency!

Thinking back to Nov. 2019, and the happy memories...I volunteered to compose music for scenes in a play called... [*Coronavirus brain fog, for the life of me, I can't think of the play.* -15 minutes later-I ask my husband-just coming home.] The music I created and recorded was for a II Act Play called *Silent Sky*, which was presented by our local Olympic Theatre Arts (OTA). It was challenging, but fun, as I was brought on board when the play was well underway. There was an exhilarating type of pressure I felt of following the script and creating appropriate music that would fit the mood required of each scene. I loved the challenge, and was able to see the show performed just before leaving for my, year in advanced planned, vacation. I composed and recorded the music created, plus a church hymn *"For the Beauty of the Earth,"* in seventeen days!

*Silent Sky* was still being performed, even as I was well on my way to a "once in a lifetime" vacation to Thailand with my sister and friends.

The following is a quick rambling summary, meant to be read fast, of some of the fun activities we did. I am sharing this summary to make a point that we did all these fun activities and so much more...And this year...nada, no trips, no nothing really in the way of travel or concerts, plays, or events!

In Bangkok we visited the Wat Pho Temple and saw the Reclining Gold Buddha (also where we received intense Thai massages); we flew to Phuket staying near Kata Noi beach, did a beach/temple tour, shopped, and dined on delicious Pad Thai and had banana Roti (dessert). I tried mangosteen, and Thailand's King of fruit Durian (stinky, but yummy-licious!) We also took a boat tour of Phi Phi islands, snorkeling in the beautiful turquoise waters (amazing iridescent fishes) and relaxed on white sandy beaches. (My screen saver paradise!) From there we flew inland to Chiang Mai where I delivered a care package to an American man from his mom. (warm fuzzies to have been the courier) We watched *The Cave*, a movie about the rescue of Thai soccer team and their coach from a flooded cave; a surreal experience as I remember watching the rescue on TV in the US the year before. We visited Elephant Rescue Park (ethically treated) where I fed, touched/hugged, and bathed elephants for the first time in my life. Fun times! Back in Bangkok, we shopped at the ICONSIAM mall, and I had an authentic Thanksgiving dinner at our hotel whilst my sister and friends dined in Chinatown. On the last day we Christmas shopped at the Chatuchak Weekend Market before flying home to Washington State, via Suvarnabhumi Airport, pronounced Suwanapume, and South Korea's, Incheon Airport. I recall someone on the flight coughing quite a bit about three rows back in the center. I wore one of my masks for air pollution, the whole way home. I felt bad for the sick person and their seat companions. (novel coronavirus?)

Nov. 17th - Dec. 3rd 2019. Seventeen days total!

Seventeen days of a lot of pictures, a whirlwind jam packed itinerary, of sensory overload, meaning I just wanted to take in all the newness of the foreign surroundings. I the "Farang" or foreigner will always treasure the memories...oh, that tropical heat... one evening as we were dining, we had a sudden downpour of... thinking of *Forest Gump* here, "big ol' fat rain." Oh, the exhilarating exotic tropical memories...fast speeding erratic Tuk-tuks (Thai taxis) ...like a distant memory now. Khob-kuhn-krab, Khob-kuhn-ka (Thank you,) to the men, lady boys and women I met in Thailand for the wonderful friendly hospitality, culture, and food, you made my/our visit to Thailand extraordinary and fun!

That was then, Nov.17th - Dec. 3rd 2019. When we finally arrived home I slept, and when I was awake it was like I had just experienced a wonderful very realistic tropical dream! I was completely wiped out! I slept a lot, off and on for nearly two weeks readjusting to our time zone, and the dark, cold, short winter days of the Pacific Northwest. Bleh! Christmas snuck up on me way too quickly. Where had the month gone? I felt oddly like I was in the *Twilight Zone*. I still needed to wrap my souvenir gifts. I was exhausted! Christmas, of course, was Thai themed. Our house was scented with the tropical flower Frangipani, (no noble fir) as one of the Reed Diffuser's cap had come loose on our Christmas tree. This was right about the time we were becoming aware...

The proverbial sh** was hitting the fan! Life, as we knew it, here and around the world, was being altered in the most mind-blowing, off-teetering way! ☹

It is near the end of Dec. 2019, Wuhan, China in Hubei Province has a mysterious respiratory virus making people seriously ill and many (understated) have lost their lives to its ensuing disease. The virus manifested presumably in a wet market, and in not the most sanitary of conditions. Pangolins and bats are thought to be the probable vectors of the new deadly virus. Some in China have a penchant for feasting on wild animals, and even domestic, sadly.

**Breaking News:** "US passes 4 million corona virus cases as pace of new infections roughly doubles." July 23rd *WP.* Dave, my husband just shared the above news with me..

Reflecting back, I remember in January watching YouTube videos about this virus in Wuhan, China and thinking we are not isolated from this virus here in the United States, I just came back from Thailand, half way around the world. People get on planes every day and travel around the world. I remember worriedly expressing to my husband in January, "I don't want to have to stay home all year!" He was taken aback, "what do you mean?' 'You won't have to stay here all year!" I replied, "People are dying, it will be here next, if it isn't already." (Oh, the foreseen prophesy of those words.)

In the following days… luggage still largely left unpacked…blur of unimaginable shocking videos coming out of China. On Jan. 23rd, Wuhan, and other cities in the Hubei Province were in lock down. There was drone footage showing haunting aerial views of what appeared to be completely desolate cities devoid of life; People in hazmat suits, masks, goggles…and the incredible feat of watching the Chinese construction workers building a massive hospital complex in just over a week's time! A page has turned in history… on the cusp of, "our new normal," here in the United States.

So, so many YouTube videos, I followed *JaYoe Nation*, Mathew Galat who would usually be cycling around the world on a recumbent trike, until the coronavirus appeared. He is an American married to a Chinese woman named Anny (nice singing voice) and they are the parents to Eva who loves dinosaurs. I watched their journey from Nimbo, China to the United States, and back to Nimbo, China again. I remember Matt talking about the ease in which they came through the airport, he said, "It was a bit too easy," even as they were about to go into a voluntary 14-day quarantine. Needless to say, that ease, was somewhat revealing as to how little prepared the United States was in the face of the novel coronavirus. His family thankfully didn't have the coronavirus, and when they returned home to Nimbo, China they were faced with temperature checks, swab testing and mandatory separate coronavirus quarantine. Matt often speaks of, "ripples" the affects we have on one another with words and actions. So true, Matt, if you ever should read this, I hope you and yours are still doing well.

I also watched a man named Hai Tang, *ErgengTV*, who documented his wife, Li Ting, an emergency room nurse's Covid-19 infection at home and in the hospital. When Li Ting was finally released I had so many tears of relief and joy for her recovery, Li Ting had a long and difficult struggle to recovery. I loved the coming home video, no Hollywood, "fake reality" the reunion was real and emotions raw. Anyone watching knew she had just been through an incredible battle for her life! The reunion with their son, Shi Tou after 74 days being apart was very touching. Shi Tou had stayed with his grandparents.

I recall another YouTuber in particular, a courageous man named Chen Qiushi, a lawyer and citizen journalist, who was determined to document all he was witnessing in Wuhan. Paraphrasing, - Chen was fearful of the virus in front of him and the Chinese Authorities behind him, but he was determined to share what he was witnessing even if he should die. - I cried then, seeing it, and just now revisiting the YouTube video, I am crying again. I have thought of him often as the coronavirus spreads its invisible, infectious deadly strain here in America and around the entire world. If I could somehow rescue Chen, I would. My heart is still wounded just to think of him. I wanted to hug him, protect him. This mama just wanted to get him out of there! It is said that he was taken into quarantine even though he didn't show any signs of having the virus, and he hasn't been seen since.

My feelings for Chen's safety just made me think about another man I couldn't rescue…

And when I heard George call for his mama… this protective mama yelled for that heartless police officer to, "Get the F off his neck, stop kneeling on him, he CAN'T BREATHE you &*% a**holes!" Tears of frustration, pain and the inhumanity of what I and the world witnessed {after the fact} just resurfaced again. R.I.P George Floyd, AKA Big Floyd. 10/14/73- 5/25/20, your life mattered, Black Lives Matter. Police Reform is happening.

I wanted to order a George Floyd mask. I went online and found masks, but when I went to place my order they were made differently, in the written description, from what the picture had illustrated. Nylon spandex being the innermost layer to a person's face, my first thought was how itchy it might be, but then also how could anyone possibly breathe with that fabric?!? I Google searched nylon spandex, low, and behold, nylon-*an unbreathable fabric*. I wrote the first review to this company telling them to, "Let America Breathe!" and sent them a screenshot about nylon spandex not being breathable…the next day I couldn't locate the ads for those masks anywhere. I remember seeing something about "price gouging" with the sale of masks. It is my hope that the company took my words to heart and pulled their ads.

I had planned to travel to Seattle to attend the peaceful march against police brutality because I felt strongly about the senseless death of George Floyd, and other victims of police brutality. I didn't go though, as my husband discouraged the notion, with this pandemic in full swing. And as things unfolded, I was somewhat relieved I wasn't victimized by the police or rabble-rousers in the melee that it unfortunately turned into. It really does say something when in the midst of a pandemic people all across America, who are supposed to be social distancing, were/are willing to protest (most wearing masks) for the sake of social justice. A wake-up call for police departments across America! George Floyd's death made Americans and the world shudder. Not to mention, other acts of blatant disregard for human life captured on police body cams and the public's cell phones. We as a nation have a responsibility to hold our police departments accountable. And as for criminals (hate groups) opportunists, stealing, looting, burning, they too should also be held accountable. "Two wrongs don't make it right." The anger of course is justified, but that righteous anger should be channeled toward positive change.

We know, without a doubt, that not every cop is a bad cop. People felt passionate in expressing their anger regarding George Floyd's death and that of other victims of police brutality. Please take a moment to read the following Facebook post: *To the people and my friends of Seattle and surrounding area. Toda*...Josh Johnson

The post can be found at *'You lost a good one': Local officers question future in law enforcement amid intense backlash, civil unrest* Q13 FOX, Seattle June 9

We need to have open discussions between police departments and the public. National Reform. How else will we find resolve? I pray Josh Johnson does not turn in his badge.

Rayshard Brooks comes to mind. Inebriated, but that aside he was very polite and cooperative. He just needed to sleep it off. The officer even originally suggested, "Just pull somewhere and take a nap..." It is too late now, he is gone. No eighth Birthday celebration with his daughter, (the next day) or any other occasion for that matter. Rayshard likely was feeling threatened and had a "fight or flight" response to the officers. The situation really should never have escalated to the point of a scuffle and Taser grab. R.I.P Rayshard Brooks, 1/3/98-6/13/20

Life is precious. If only more people would respect and believe that. Life is precious. Life is a gift. We want to live, we want to breathe, and we want to be healthy and happy. Breonna Taylor died tragically after a "No knock warrant." Her boyfriend who is licensed to carry had aimed low so as not to kill the intruder(s) but to send a clear message that he was protecting his home and loved ones. 6/5/93-3/13/20, an EMT she worked the Frontline- R.I.P Breonna Taylor. She saved lives she was a heroine. "No knock warrants" are becoming a thing of the past.

Let's be heroes and heroines too! People are wearing masks because there is legitimate reason to be fearful, and because they care about themselves and others.

**Please, America wear your masks.**

It has been cathartic to express my thoughts and feelings with you the reader. Seven months into it now. 18 -22 months they say...I have been praying right along with you for an effective vaccine. I've been doing the "Staying home, to stay healthy," As Governor Jay Inslee mandated back in March. No exciting trips for me this year. I have been a homebody for seven months! We are in Phase 2 here in our neck of the woods, but technically I am still in Phase 1. Why? The virus is deadly and seemingly determined to infect people everywhere. It has taken awhile for some to come around and realize the seriousness of this novel coronavirus. It isn't a hoax, farce, or conspiracy! It is the real deal! Washington State announced on January 21st, the first official confirmed case in Snohomish County- he survived. And I too survived Swine Flu in 2009. So I am on a mission, to help all of us to not only survive, but thrive in this crazy world pandemic year of 2020!

The following exercises were created to give visual perspectives of Covid-19 as if it were infecting your state and your state alone! That is, Covid-19 US population deceased **concentrated** into one specific state, and that specific state being where you reside. The task ahead will give a completed exercise, and one to continue if you are inclined to do so. When I did the exercises, I felt angry, (so many still hoo-hawing.) Anger is also a natural response to fear, followed by sadness, and lastly resolve. A resolve to, "bring it home" for others. A sense of urgency came over me to share this VisualPerspective.

I want for YOU to be as **determined** as I am in doing all that **you can** to **avoid becoming infected** with Covid-19. How? By making the "personal freedom" sacrifices necessary to flatten the curve! Those residing in the United States of America and her US Territories masked, hands clean and standing 6' apart in a UNITED front against this invisible deadly enemy. -True Patriotism, defined.

We got this, America! Let's protect one another. Thank you, President Donald J. Trump on July 11, 2020 you finally decided to wear a mask. At last, you've led our nation by example.

In 100 days, America, we vote! Dear Mr. President voting by mail is the safest and most protective way to keep our United States in the direction of flattening the curve. Voting by mail, **will** save LIVES!

The SARS-CoV-2 novel coronavirus, Covid-19 should never have become a political issue. It is, however, everyone's common enemy, so no matter your political affiliation, Democrat, Republican, Independent, and or of no affiliation at all, we **need** to treat it as such! We may not agree on everything. We can agree to disagree on political viewpoints. But this Covid-19 is a whole other ball game!

(Which, by the way, most sports fans are missing) Covid-19 is
not a hoax! Understand? Capeesh? So let's get to it!

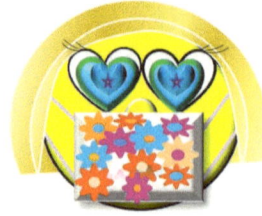

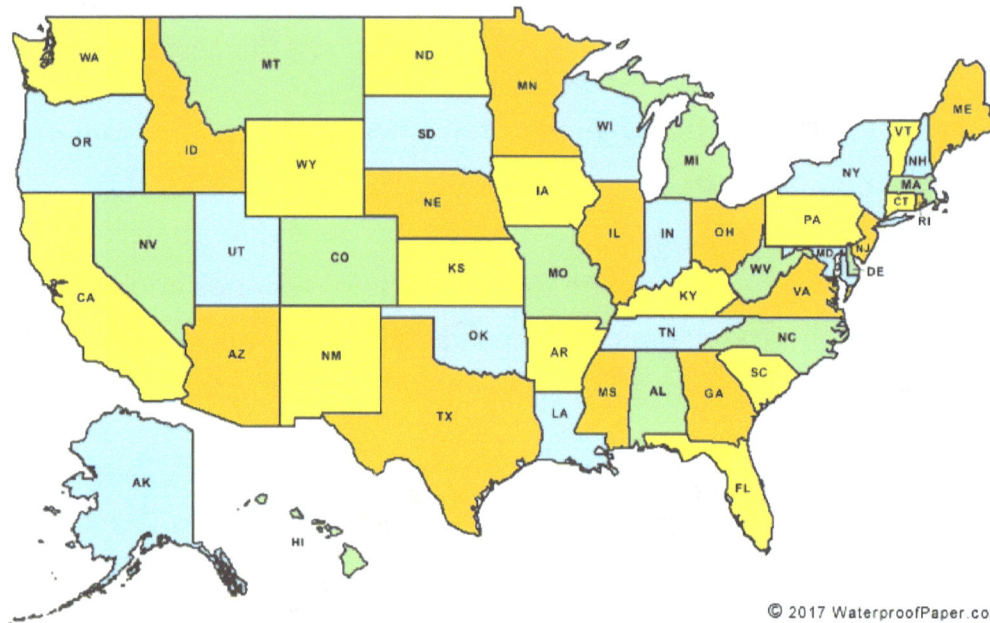

© 2017 WaterproofPaper.com

**VisualPerspective, Getting Started:** Covid-19 deceased in the USA, in relation to your State of_____and Counties within.

Supplies: Worksheets provided in the back of this book, pencil, blue pen, red gel pen, highlight marker, computer/smartphone/calculator, and printer.

1. Go to ncov2019.live, either, "Jump to Region" USA or beyond **Quick Facts** for the World, you will see under TOTAL ☆ United States, (1st on the list of countries.) In green, are confirmed Covid-19. In red, are deceased - God rest their souls. - Write down on your worksheet(s) the TOTAL deceased in the USA, then indicate today's date and time. Close out of site, or add page.

2. Key in, **free printable maps**, on your search bar. It will bring up *Images* (of maps) and just below them you'll see the following: **Free Printable Maps | World, USA, State, City, County – Waterproof Paper** Easy to print maps. Download and print...

3. Click on the state where you live. (X out of any ads) print **2 copies** of, **Your State** County Map with County Names *Please print black and white version. Close out of site.

4. Key in: your state name-washington-demographics.com Scroll down, past state information and ads, until you see **State's Counties by Population.** Open (next to eyeball👁) **See all your State Counties by Population.** Find the County of the city, town, or community where you live. Write the estimated population of your county (**in blue**) under the corresponding county on your state map. If your county appears small you may draw an arrow to the outer margin and then write your population (**in blue**) If uncertain of your home county, key in, what county is_____town, city, or community in? Google will bring up your county. Include today's date and **asterisk. ***

💜 **Your Population   is Less than...**

1. Is the estimated census population of your county **less** than Covid-19 deceased for all of the United States today? If **yes**, trace your county in red; If you haven't already, write your county population under your county name or in the margin, (**in blue**) and date. (If **no**, skip 2-5)

2. Now going back to the web page **ncov2019.live** Coronavirus Dashboard, check to see, has the total US deceased number of Covid-19 increased? If **yes**, write down this new total of Covid-19 deceased for the United States, again noting today's date, and current time. Subtract your County's population from the USA deceased total.

   **Example:** 143,440 Total Deceased in US, **7/19**, 9:20 AM

            - 22,425 Population of <u>Home County</u>

            **121,015** US Deceased Difference

   **VisualPerspective:** All of your home <u>Name of County</u>, _____ and the US difference_____ **deceased**. Shocking, to say the least!

3. Take a look at the list of counties for your, **state name-demographics.com** How many counties are there all together in the state you reside?_____Counties altogether. Counties are numbered in the order from the largest populated county down to the least populated county.

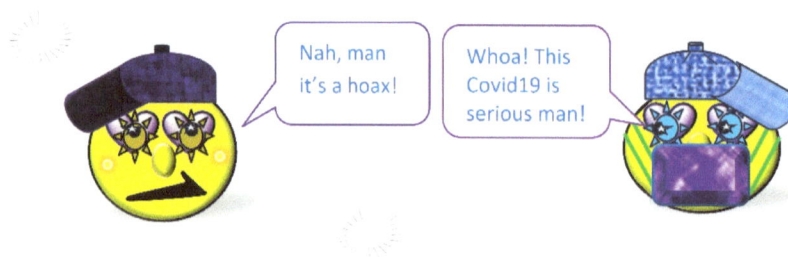

4. Taking another look at your list of counties go to the least populated county, it will be the last numbered county for your state. **Example:** Ranked, 1 for most populated county down 39 for least populated county.

   The least populated county should be **less** than the US Deceased Difference of your home county.

   Subtract the population of the county, and move up to the next county population in line. (ex. 39, 38, 37...) Please write neatly, County name next to population amount being subtracted and ranked number; locate and trace the county on your state map, in red and then in blue the population amount corresponding with the county either in the County itself, or the margin.

   > **Example:** 143,440 Total Deceased in US, **7/19**, 9:20 AM
   > - 22,425 Population of <u>Home County</u>
   > 121,015 US Deceased Difference
   > -   2,225   Population of <u>Least Pop. Name County</u>
   > 118,790   US Deceased Difference
   > -   4,488   Population of <u>Up the line, Name County</u>

   So on and so forth...

5. Continue subtracting the county populations as you move up the line, until the US Deceased Difference is **less** than the population of the county next in line. <mark>Highlight</mark> the remaining US Deceased Difference and date.

   **Example:** <mark>9,939 US Deceased Remaining, **7/19**</mark>

23

💗**Your Population    is Less than... continued**

**VisualPerspective:** How many counties in Your State were **totally deceased**?_____Write it down and indicate, Deceased. Let that sink in for a moment... Imagine everyone in your own county--- that's cities, towns, and communities--- WIPED out countywide! An invisible deadly, corona virus, Covid-19 has totally taken out the entire population of your county! That is ALL the people living (past tense) in your hometown and all the neighboring cities, towns, and communities of your particular county. Furthermore, same goes for ALL the other counties, and their cities, towns, and communities. DEAD! It is devastating to see! **Note:** The US Deceased Remaining <mark>highlighted</mark> from the previous page will be used for another exercise later.

We have the power to alter Covid-19's deadly onslaught! We as a nation can band together against SARS-CoV-2 novel coronavirus that can lead to Covid-19 respiratory illness, and ultimately for some death.

We together can flatten the curve! ⟶

Skip, 💗 **Your Population is Greater than...** as it doesn't apply to you.

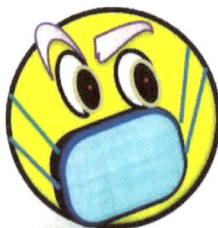

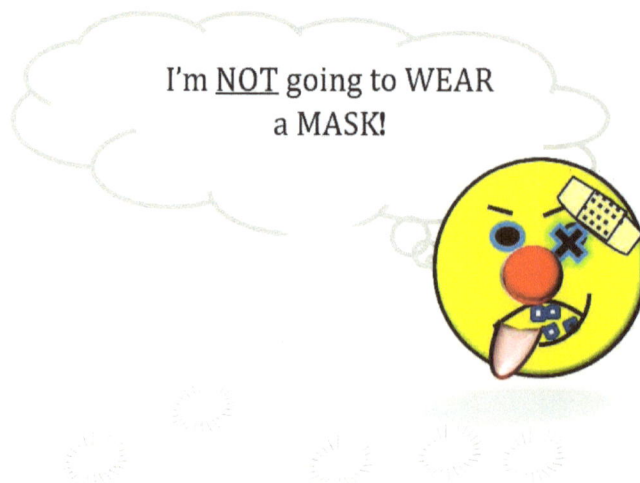

I'm <u>NOT</u> going to WEAR a MASK!

💜Your Population   is Greater than...

1. The population of your county is greater than the amount of Covid-19 deceased in the United States. Before we proceed, check **ncov2019.live** has the total US deceased number of Covid-19 increased? If **yes**, write down this new total of Covid-19 deceased for the United States, again noting today's date, and current time.

2. Now take a look at the list of counties for your **state name-demographics.com** How many counties are there all together in the state you reside?_____Counties altogether. Counties are numbered in the order from the largest populated county down to the least populated county.

3. Determine what would be the deceased percentage amount of the Total US deceased as it relates to the Greater population of the <u>Home County</u>, where you reside. Write the_____% amount **in red** on your county.

   **Example:** 143,440 Deceased in US, **7/19**, 9:20 AM

   ÷ <u>229,247</u> Population, <u>Home County</u>
   0.62570066 X 100= **62.5%** Deceased, **7/19**

25

4. How many people are still alive in your county? Take the population of your home county and subtract the total deceased in the US following the example below. Write the amount living_____ **in blue** on your worksheet(s).

**Example:**  229, 247 Population, <u>Home County</u>

-    <u>143,440</u> Total Deceased in US, **7/19**, 9:20 AM

**85,807**  Difference still Alive!

**VisualPerspective:** Let the percentage____**%** sink in for a moment. How did your <u>Home County</u> look? Was the deceased population less than half? Was the deceased population over half of the population deceased? It is difficult to fathom, but that would be the reality if the Covid-19 deaths for the United States were concentrated into the State County where you reside. And yet, hopefully many are still alive!

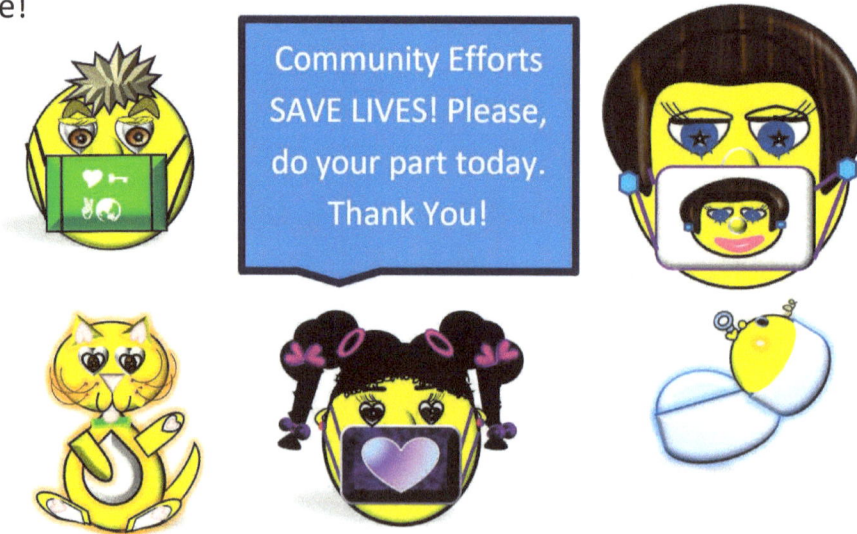

Community Efforts SAVE LIVES! Please, do your part today. Thank You!

**WE have the POWER to…** ─────────➔

Each one of us has the power to protect ourselves and our loved ones. We currently do not have a vaccine for Covid-19 or treatment that leads to a cure. However, per **ncov2019.live.com** there are currently 155 vaccines in development. (*156 vaccines) This is very promising. Note: Site updates information daily. This coronavirus is novel, meaning it hasn't previously been identified. It is a deadly strain of virus that can spread asymptomatically, meaning a person may not show symptoms and yet will still be contagious. Not everyone infected dies. However, there is no point in taking any chances! Risky behavior (not wearing a mask) could kill you, and or your loved ones. As unintentional as it might be, you could also be responsible for the death of friends, family, strangers, and your favorite barber or beautician. Period! And a few expletives *&$% to boot!

Then there are unsung heroes, Frontline workers, deemed Essential, for me personally that means: Propane Technicians, Fuel Deliverers (husband, 1st born son, & nephew), Car maintenance (2nd born son), Personal Banker (1st born son's girlfriend), Big-Box Store Cap II (2nd born son's girlfriend), Pharmacist, Pharmacy Techs, (sister), Communications Technician (brother), Car Wash Manager (brother's girlfriend, phase 2) Government DOD (sister, & her boyfriend), Waste Management (nephew), Mailperson (niece, & her boyfriend), Wine Manager (niece), Restaurant/Barista (niece)…if anyone of my loved ones became ill with Covid-19 they would be dependent on the Essential Frontline, Nurses and Doctors, who are giving their ALL each day to try to save Covid-19 patients' and regular patients' lives! They are doing this, at times with limited supplies of, personal protective equipment (PPE) ventilators/oxygen and or available beds. And astoundingly, they will take care of you whether you were cooperative in wearing your masks or not! -The implications of such irresponsible behavior…they are putting their own lives on the line! It bodes well to reiterate we are in a World Pandemic, National Emergency!

These Doctors and nurses are doing the best they can to treat patients with Covid-19; a virus strain that is stealthy in its infectious nature, benign for some and deadly for others. They are also providing palliative care for those in the throes of death, because family and friends cannot be there, as PPE is limited, and the possible <u>risk</u> of exposure to the SARS-CoV-2. Speaking of- <u>risks</u>- Frontline Custodians sterilize patient's rooms. Courageous heroes, each and every one! But no matter how brave our heroes and heroines are, they are <u>only human</u> and can only handle so much! If Hospitals are inundated and overwhelmed with patients, the quality of care given may be sacrificed. (Curve goes up.)

<u>Flattening the</u> curve- OUR lives may just depend on it!!!

I feel it important to point out the obvious, not everyone employed is considered, an "Essential" worker in Phase 1. "Essential," probably isn't the greatest choice of words to describe which employees are necessary for the function of society. As everyone's job is <u>Essential</u> in the manner of bringing home the bacon, mortgage payments, rent, food, clothes, etc. It is not lost on me that my husband has had steady employment throughout this pandemic. (blue collar America.) It is a risk though each time he and other, "essential" workers leave their homes for work- Most businesses are taking stricter measures for employees' health. Wearing masks, (w/labor intensive jobs) hasn't been easy to do, however, it is necessary for the protection of one's self and others. Currently, with the easing of Phase 2, it is riskier still, as professions such as Beautician, Nail Technician are "up close and personal." (Each state's mandates are different) UGH! Health officials and government officials are doing what they can to look out for the health and safety of the citizens of their individual states. (Depending on where you live) I understand and empathize with the difficult situation many people are currently in. Unemployment/Stimulus Checks are temporary fixes. I pray we get some semblance of normalcy back sooner than later.

We're, "all in the same boat" with different circumstances and impositions. Wait, do we want to be in the same boat? i.e. Cruise Ships :-O

Our Nitro Circus Live Tour, Fri- May 8, 2020 -7:00 PM at the Evergreen Speedway in Monroe, WA, My Big Kahuna Christmas present for my husband and sons, has been postponed due to this Pandemic. It is what it is!

We as a nation should be determined to fight this,... #@&*% invisible enemy!!!

Are you with me on this?

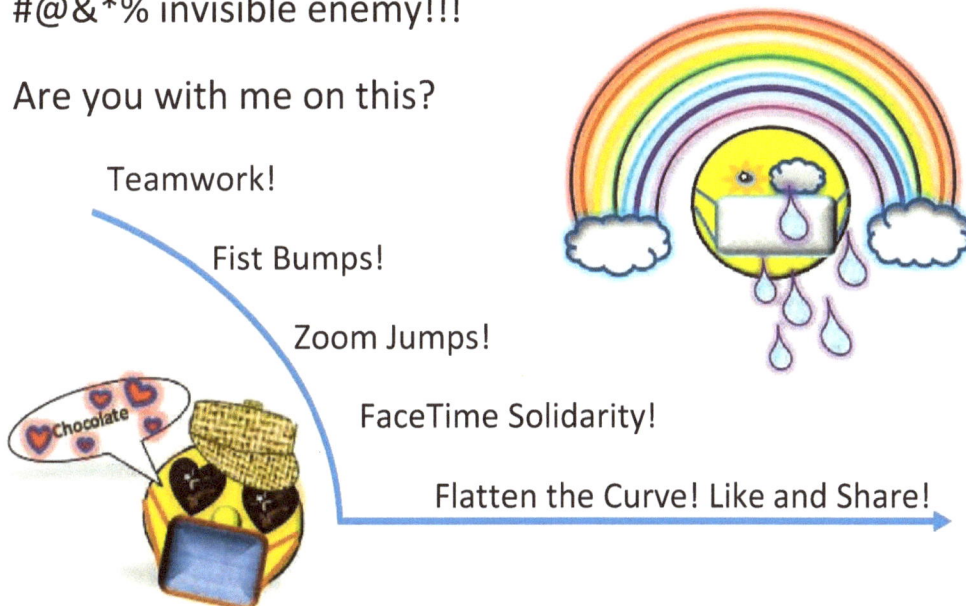

Teamwork!

Fist Bumps!

Zoom Jumps!

FaceTime Solidarity!

Flatten the Curve! Like and Share!

What's on Netflix tonight? I love the South Korean Drama with Subtitles, called _Chocolate_. A romantic love story, "first loves" meet as adults. The story line and beautiful heart- touching music pulled at my husband's and my heartstrings. Just beautiful, as you might guess, I am listening to it now. "Just look for you" Artist Ailee

I would be remiss if I didn't mention a few of the awesome YouTubers making the world smile, laugh and even have a good cry. When the pandemic stress is getting to be too much! **YouTubers:** The Holderness Family, Chris Mann, The Kiffness, Julie Nolke, (Canadian neighbor) Trey Kennedy, and for beautiful duets the father and daughter Mat and Savana Shaw, _"The Prayer."_ 💜

💗Your Population   Both Less than and Greater than…

1. **Set your first state and county map aside**, but save: Let's now revisit the state demographic site. Key in your **state-demographics.com**

   **\* Second copy of Map with State and Counties…**

   Referencing your state's county populations, place a **red X** for **every county** population that is **less** than the deceased total of US Population. Check for latest stats at **ncov2019.live** Allow your mind the VisualPerspective of considering **ALL of these lives** in each of these counties as **deceased**. Depending on your state's population, the map could look disheartening for sure. Like a lottery ticket you know is a loser. How many counties were completely deceased? Write the number in the margin of your map. You may opt to trace each of the exed **X** counties for visual impact.

2. Write down **in blue** all of the remaining county populations. Divide each one of the county populations into the total deceased in the US to determine the **%** percentage of deaths for each county. Then write the____**%** in each corresponding counties **in red**.

   **Example:** 143,440 Total Deceased in US, **7/19**, 9:20 AM

   ÷ 488,241 Population of <u>Large Populated County</u>

   0.29378934 X 100= **29.3%** Deceased

3. Who is still alive?!? How many are still living in each of the remaining counties with **%** percentages of deceased? Take the population for each county and subtract the deceased in the US as noted following the **example on the next page**. Write the difference still alive in each corresponding counties **in blue**.

31

💗**Your Population   Less than and Greater than… continued**

**After that exercise, we need some good news! I am hopeful.**

**Example:** 488,241 Large Population of- <u>County Name</u>

  -<u>143,440</u> Total Deceased in US, **7/19**, 9:20 AM

  **344,801**   Difference Alive!


4.  Add **ALL**, still alive differences, from the remaining counties.

   **Example: Difference Alive + Difference Alive + Difference Alive + Difference Alive + Difference Alive + Difference Alive + Difference Alive = *Hope Several* Million People Still Alive!**


**VisualPerspective:** Seeing a lot of **red X's**- without a doubt. Hopefully your state has larger populated counties with **blue** still very much alive! How did your state do?

All of OUR efforts here in the United States, US Territories and Countries around the world are what is going to make a positive difference in this, let's just face it, "New Normal." Our efforts will help flatten the curve, and relieve our frontline nurses and doctors from becoming overwhelmed with too many patients. If anyone of us happened to get Covid-19 and were hospitalized, we would want to receive the best care we could possibly get. We would want a bed available, and as admitted patients, if we needed oxygen supplementation, we would want it to be readily available. Furthermore, if our infection became really serious, we would want to have the option of being intubated with a ventilator, which supports breathing (induced coma). It cannot be emphasized enough, that Doctors should **not** be placed in the uncomfortable position of determining which one of us receives oxygen and or ventilator. The decisions made could mean life or death. There are hospitals across the United States that have already experienced being stretched to their limits.

## STOP!

You need not take anything a step further. I believe the

VisualPerspective has definitely been obtained.

💗 **Your Population** ☺**k**

**Taking this VisualPerspective a Step Further...**

In perspective, it may seem morbid to carry on keeping track of the coronavirus Covid-19. However, if you find this Covid-19 VisualPerspective is something you would want to continue doing, by all means continue. Let's hope that more state counties remain untraced, rather than traced. That would be exciting news, as it would reveal we are WINNING the battle against Covid-19! In other words, more LIVES saved! If we do our part to stay healthy; wear our masks, wash hands frequently, maintain social distancing of at least 6' from other people especially outside our immediate, "hubs" we can make a positive difference. We've got this! It's an inconvenience but relatively EASY to do!

**\*VisualPerspective: Using your <u>first map</u>** the exercise will continue to serve as a visual reminder of where America stands on flattening the curve. Its' purpose is to show the impact Covid-19 is having on America as a whole, but condensed into one state, -**<u>Your State specifically</u>**.

**Track:** 💗 **Your Population    is Less than... First map**

**A Review:** You indicated your county population, dated, and asterisked * it on your map and traced your county in red. You were able to subtract the **least populated county** from the Difference of your Home County population, subtracted from the Total US Deceased Population.

You were likely able to further subtract other smaller populated counties in your state, coming up the list from least populated on up. **For example:** 39, 38, 37... 32 County numbers by population. You subsequently traced each county in red, and noted the population for each county, in blue.

You continued to move up the line and subtract until the **US difference could no longer subtract**, as it was **less** than the next county up the line.

The US Deceased, remaining, was <mark>highlighted</mark> and dated.

Previous example

Example: <mark>9,939 US Deceased Remaining, **7/19**</mark>

**Hashtags**: #wearadamnmask, #masketorcasket, #stayhome, #safedistance... 6' apart is a good place to start!

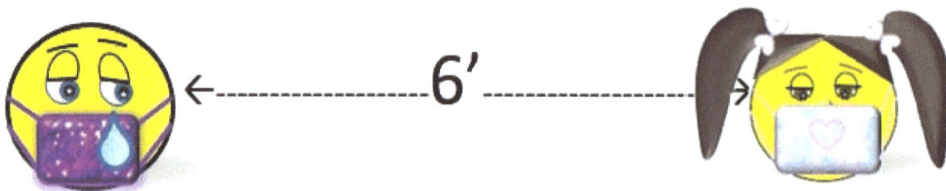

**YouTube:** Luke Coombs, *Six feet Apart* (Lyric Video) 5.4M views

You may track week to week; month to month, to the day or date- Any deceased difference remaining, should be <mark>highlighted</mark> and dated, for the following week or month that you track.

**Example:** *Not tempting fate*  Total Deceased in US, **7/26**, time

        -<u>143,440</u>    Total Deceased in US, **7/19**, 9:20 AM

        *Hope Diff. not many*    Deceased Difference **7/26**

<mark>        + <u>9,939</u>     US Deceased Diff. Remaining, **7/19**</mark>

        *\*Hope Total not many*    Deceased Total **7/26**

        *- <u>Next County Population</u>*    Name of County, Date

\*Continue to subtract if the US total difference is **more** than the *Next County up*, otherwise <mark>Highlight,</mark> and save to track for the following week, and or month to the date. I pray you won't have to subtract each time.

**Breaking News:** July 21, 2020, "US reports more than 1,000 coronavirus deaths in a day for the first time since early June" *WP*

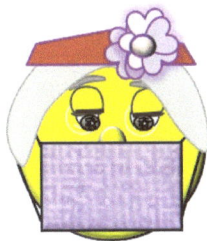

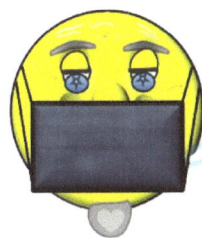

Please wear a Mask, that's ALL we ask.

**Track:** 💗 **Your Population    is Greater than... First map**

**A Review:** Your estimated census population for your <u>Home County</u> was greater than the deceased number for all the United States. You wrote the estimated county population for your Home County, dated, **asterisked***it on your map, traced your county **in red**, and noted the percentage_____ **%** You also subtracted the Total US deceased from your county population to determine how many were still living. You then indicated **in blue**, the Difference still alive on your worksheet(s). Below are the previous examples.

<br>

**Example:** 143,440 Deceased in US, **7/19**, 9:20 AM

÷ <u>229,247</u> Population, <u>Home County</u>

==0.62570066 X 100 = **62.5%** US Deceased Difference, **7/19**==

<br>

**Example:** 229, 247 Population, <u>Home County</u>

-<u>143,440</u> Total Deceased in US, **7/19**, 9:20 AM

**85,807**  Difference Alive!

<br>

(I started wearing masks early-on in March. I remember some looked at me with admiration, thinking perhaps I was a caregiver, nurse, or a physician; still others looked at me like I was a complete idiot. (Rude comments) and then others had looks of envy. (Wishing they had a mask too) I remember going to our local grocer and a produce guy and I were the only ones wearing masks. Now, everyone is masked in this grocery store including the deli ladies who snickered at me.)

**Track: 💗 Your Population   is Greater than... continued**

1. Continue to track your percentages of deceased for your Home County until your county is **100%** deceased, or you cannot bear to keep track any longer. You may write the **percentages %** directly on your county map or separately on the worksheets.

   I want to encourage you to write the living difference on your worksheet in the back, **in blue**.

   **Example:** *Not tempting Fate* Deceased in US, **7/26**, Date, Time

   $\div$ <u>229,247</u>   Population, <u>Home County</u>

   *Percentage____%*   US Deceased Difference, **7/26**

   *So on and so forth...*

   **Example:**        229, 247   Population, <u>Home County</u>

   - <u>Not tempting Fate</u>   Total Deceased in US, **7/26**, Date

   **Your Population**   Difference Alive!

   *So on and so forth...until*

2. If your population becomes 100% deceased, heaven forbid, you'll subtract from the total US deceased and highlight the US Difference. See example on the following page.

**Track: 💗 Your Population is Greater than... continued**

**Example:** *Not tempting fate* Total Deceased in US, Date, Time

        -229,247        100% Deceased <u>Home County,</u> Date

        <mark>*US Difference*</mark>        US Deceased Difference, Date, Time

3. Starting with the least populated county in your state. Is the least populated county less than the US Deceased difference? If **yes**, go ahead and subtract that county's population, then write the county's population **in blue** under county name on your map and trace county it **in red.** They are now deceased. <mark>Highlight</mark> and write date for the difference remaining. Note: There could be more than one county subtracted. Hopefully not.

**Example:** <mark>*US Difference*</mark>    US Deceased Difference, Date, Time

        - 2,225      Population of <u>Least Pop. County</u>

        <mark>*US Difference*</mark>    US Deceased Difference, Date

Any US Difference remaining that cannot subtract the next county in line, will be <mark>highlighted</mark> and added to the US Total deceased for the following week; or month, to the day or date, depending on what you've chosen to do.

**Track:** 💗 **Your Population is Greater than... continued**

**Example:** <mark>*US Difference*</mark>   Deceased in the US Difference, Date

+ *Not tempting fate* Total deceased in the US, Date, Time

*Hope not many*    Deceased, Date

-*Closest to deceased difference* Population of <u>Name County,</u> Date

<mark>*Difference*</mark>            US Deceased Diff. Remaining, Date

4. If the answer was **no,** continue to track weekly or monthly until the US Deceased Difference Remaining plus the new total can subtract the next county line **ex.** 39, 38, 37, and so on...

I hope it never does.

The <mark>*Difference*</mark> is considered Remaining; it means there wasn't a county with a population the same or less than the <mark>*Difference*</mark> *to subtract.*

Keep up your efforts wearing your masks. We can and will flatten the curve!

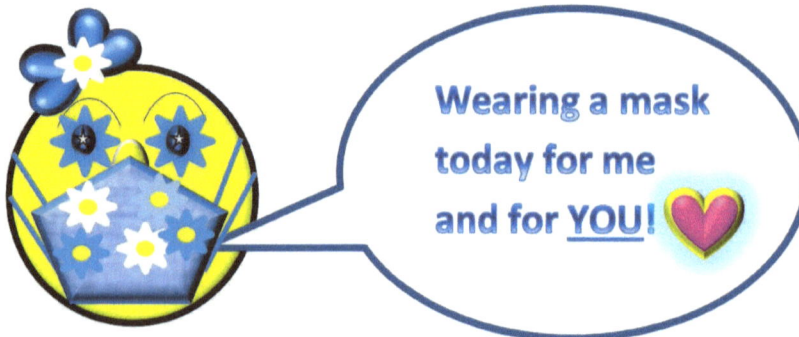

Wearing a mask today for me and for YOU! 💗

**Seven Months into this**…

It has been seven months, as I write this, the year is over half over. Red Rover, Red Rover…I've spent entire days in my nightgown, today a prime example. I've written letters to my husband's Operations Manager, requesting action to protect the employees, and to our Governor, Jay Inslee, about the Life Care nursing home and him still allowing visitors, (it only takes one person) because he didn't want to take what he called "draconian" measures, and Governor Andrew Cuomo of, New York about YouTube videos of disturbing testimonials from nurses in overwhelmed hospitals. I wrote Comic Con Representatives when they were considering carrying on with, the show, back in March. I wrote the President of our local College, on behalf of my son, a student, as school was still in session, and to our local Health Officer, Dr. Unthank and others…It isn't that I've been completely homebound, numb sitting in a corner, feeling sorry for myself and others, I've been proactive in expressing genuine concerns that can and do affect public health and safety.

I definitely have curtailed the activities I usually would be doing. No Zumba or swimming at the YMCA, even before it was closed; nor really visiting friends; also shopping trips into town- have been limited- to food shopping and other hygiene essentials; I usually have at least three new pair of sandals by now, and a few new outfits for summer. I've both cleaned and neglected my home. I took down all the curtains washed and ironed them; as I said earlier, I've been, "Staying home, to Stay Healthy." I cleaned and oiled all of our cabinets. (That took four days). It feels like one day just rolls into the next. Some days are more ambitious than others. It is the mundane tasks. - Sorting and cleaning out the spice drawer; getting rid of expired, outdated foods, i.e. baking powder, flour, condiments, and detailing our fridge. My husband cleaned our dryer vent and duct work, and behind the fridge. I recommend everyone do this as cleaning will prevent possible fires from built up lint or pet fur.

My sister, a Frontline worker, had borrowed my car because hers was in the shop, she returned it detailed and vacuumed inside and out! I didn't realize it for two weeks! That is how long it took for me to go anywhere again. Needless to say, I thanked her for detailing my car. She probably wondered what took me so long to acknowledge her. I've been taking walks nearby and bringing bubbles with me. It is meditative. I listen to the rustling of leaves in the trees as the afternoon wind picks up, the birds and the persistent tinnitus in my right ear. (I pretend that I am hearing cicadas.) I am feeling a little kooky. My rosacea flares and I'm actually grateful to have a mask, oddly enough, as it hides the redness. I've sewn several masks and given them away, and have had days where I can't find the ambition to do much of anything. The enormity of lost lives due to this pandemic weighs me down.

I recently visited a dear friend, each of us wearing our masks and keeping a, "strangers' distance" between us, it was a condolence visit. My friend's dad had passed from, you guessed it, Covid-19. God rest your soul Alejandro. He's Bolivian, was living in Bolivia, South America, but he might as well have been living just down the street, as the novel coronavirus has managed to spread itself all around the world. My husband's friend Scottie has been recovering from Covid-19. He lives in Oklahoma, a hotspot. He just recently told my husband, via text, because it was too difficult for him to talk, "You don't want to get this shit, man take every precaution!"- I was tested myself. My test results were negative. I purchased an expensive antigen test, and printed the voucher, but I still have yet to travel off the Peninsula to a clinic in Kitsap County. It is quite the distance, but I want to know if I have the antibodies.

I cannot recall exactly when, these past months have blended one into another, maybe it was in January or March; I was having pneumonia-like crackling in my chest, at night when I breathed. I remember googling, "death rattle" not knowing what was causing it. I remember experiencing tightness in my chest, and feeling as if I was gasping for air whenever my son or husband upset me. I've had extreme unexplained migraines, and bouts of diarrhea that still persist to this day. (TMI, I know) I was also experiencing temperature fluctuations, 99.8°- 100° was it a fever or menopause? I remember a day when we were looking for a travel trailer for my son and his girlfriend, temporary living quarters, as our place is very cozy, (long winded) just to say, I had this incredible muscle pain in my lower back, hips and legs, I could barely walk, it was the oddest thing. Granted I've had both hips replaced, but it was as if I needed surgery all over again. Was it novel coronavirus? I don't know. I didn't lose my sense of taste or smell, so maybe not.

In some way or another, I am certain your life has echoed mine. Each of us feeling stir crazy. Gift cards unused, movie vouchers, concerts cancelled or postponed. Summer Vacations are most certainly now going to be, "Stay Cations!"

My feelings run the gamut. I've tried to stay upbeat with uplifting music like, *Happy* Pharrell Williams, *Good Morning* Mandisa and other uplifting joyful music, dancing, singing and yet I haven't really played my piano, like at all. I love piano! The feelings of profound sadness creeps in as the enormity of lives lost this year... *"Girl you better try to have fun..."*

Randomly singing Sinead O'Connor's, *Nothing Compares 2 U...* And now I know part ways why- My opening paragraph- "Seven months..." and [*seven hours*] *15 days.* Lol *"All the flowers that you planted Mama...'* tears streaming, *'Nothing compares to you..."*

And "singing" of flowers, ironically, last fall I planted bags of bulbs for spring blooms. My beds were colorful and fit for the Easter Bunny! –fragrant with hyacinth and daffodils, tulips and later Allium which are now spent, and as my mom has pointed out look like Covid-19 being spherical in shape. I managed to do my four hanging baskets this year; the beds are virtually empty even with the addition of an automatic watering system, I couldn't bring myself to purchase the geraniums, or clumping lobelia that I normally would. I did however purchase two blueberry bushes, three tomato plants, and a loganberry, still in pots from a farm stand. All I have are my baskets, climbing roses, the perennials and Hollyhocks that I planted in the spring of 2019. Hollyhocks are biannual, meaning the first year is growth, second year blooms. I got the seeds from a sweet lady who works at the Hoover Dam Museum in Boulder City, Nevada. The seeds stem from the original Hollyhocks in the 1930's.-Pink flowers on long stalks, just now blooming, are the backdrop of my bare beds. We were on a Spring Break vacation in Las Vegas, not to gamble, rather there for shows, Michael Jackson impersonator, Santana Jackson, MJ Live, Cirque du Soleil O, Terry Wayne Fator the American ventriloquist, the Titanic Exhibit (for me personally) … And the best part for my guys,  pre-planned dirt bike rides. Christmas Kahuna! I spent the morning in Boulder City, perusing the Antique shops, enjoying the heat of the desert and local fauna. I had breakfast at the Coffee Cup Café the locals raved about and then went to the museum to learn about the construction of the Hoover Dam. No one rushing me, it was nice to experience a different city, and vibe from my own. The next day we drove back from Vegas and took a Lake Mead paddle boat tour to see the massive Hoover Dam I'd just learned about. It is amazing what mankind can do when they set their minds to it. Let me repeat, it is amazing what mankind can do when they <u>set their minds to it!</u>  If men could build a massive dam, we should, at the minimum, wear a damn mask!!! Honestly, it shouldn't even be an issue for anyone at this point. Just about everyone knows someone directly affected by Covid-19, or who has died.

I wish I could understand the mindset of those ignoring the reality of the pandemic. Part of it, I think, is that many have been misinformed, or are following only a narrative that sugarcoats, and grossly underestimates the tenacity of the virus. Conspiracy theories abound, early on the misguidance of certain news broadcasters, aka Fox News. To their credit, they're wrapping their heads around it now. Certain leanings often tout, "Fake news" it can be difficult for some to know exactly what is what. In this information age, we've got news at our fingertips, live footage from all around the world. And the algorithms of searches made don't seem to deter or persuade the wayward viewer in the direction of actual science based facts. In other words, some are spoon feeding, "gobbly-gook" to themselves and aren't even aware of it. The point is we should keep seeking truth, knowledge, and understanding about this novel coronavirus. We need to be willing to analyze, reflect, and ask the difficult questions. We need to try to see and understand one another's perspectives, and to do so without pushing the other person away. I've been keeping it real with you, the reader. I may not be the brightest turnip, (smartest dummy) but I am without a doubt certain that this pandemic is serious and real.

There are those who seem to think they don't need to wear a mask because of their faith, "God will protect them." Remember the old saying, "God helps those, who help themselves." That definitely applies to the common sense measures we are/should be adhering to. Then you have folks saying, "If it's my time to go..."

BS, those words couldn't be more selfish! My response, "Don't take me with you." The virus spreads person to person, via water droplets in our spit- "micro-particles" invisible like the virus- Forceful sneezing, singing, shouting, coughing, and even just talking can cause it to spread.

I would encourage you to watch the following video.

**YouTube**: "COVID-19: See How Coronavirus Infection Spread When You Sneeze Or Cough." Apr. 8, 2020 *Indiatimes*

If what you read, view, and listen to won't sink in, I am at a loss, the music alone speaks volumes.

**More Breaking News:** "UNPROTECTED 40 Worshippers Infected With COVID-19 After Alabama Revival Congregants at the event were not required to wear masks." July 26, 2020 *Daily Beast*

**Again down Memory Lane for me, 2019 …**

Last year was jammed packed with activity and trips. My niece graduated from H.S. we pony backed her mom's promised trip to Maui. I loved shopping in Lahaina with my family. We snorkeled at Napili Beach, and I came face to face with a turtle. A man on the beach offered to help me with my fins as I was struggling to put them on in the ocean current. As it turns out he moved to Maui from Forks, WA. [*Remember* the movie *Twilight*? Edward, and Bella. I had the bright idea, but didn't follow-through, to bend the center prongs of "forks" to make the fork look like vampire teeth.] I absolutely love Maui! Half of our party left Maui on 4th of July, myself included, (son's birthday ☺ the next day) the following week Maui was on fire. I cried. It is such a beautiful island. I cried also because these fires are happening more, and more frequently. I am thinking of California and the Santa Anna winds so prevalent. Ripe conditions in the summer-time. The town of Paradise comes to mind, terrible devastation. And now once again Maui is battling fires in July 2020.

I recently was looking for the latest on Covid-19 in regard to travelling to Maui. Apparently if you are tested 72 hours in advance for Coronavirus and are negative, with proof, you can vacation there. It sounds tempting. Five hours on the plane is my only deterrent. It doesn't matter if there is an empty seat spacing apart, all passengers wearing masks, or how sterile, right now it is just too risky! Of course that is my personal opinion, but honestly any confined space with strangers, even masked strangers, removing their masks to eat and drink, would be compromising. It is a no brainer. I felt bad for those who went to Hawaii earlier and had to spend 14 days quarantining. As expensive, as it is to travel. Fortunately, certain Airlines are giving out vouchers for tickets if people were unable to travel due to the pandemic. My son and his girlfriend have had to postpone their trip and have vouchers for later.

I remember massive fires in the Amazon and Australia...wishing I could save all the Koala bears and Kangaroos...I remember being about 40 pounds lighter, wishing I had it together. I was so much more together then, than I am now, in terms of my weight and healthier food choices. And then one of America's favorite actors, (mine included) Tom Hanks and his wife Rita Wilson became infected and got Covid-19. They were set to make a movie in Australia at the time. On March 11, 2020, he and his wife made the announcement – The NBA about the same time suspended their season.

Covid-19, is an elaborate hoax?!? It's a farce! Just a flu! Not. It will go away come November some claim. One can hope. All of us wish it would go away right now! I wish by some anomaly that the virus would find "bug zappers" more appealing than people; drawn in by the alluring light and ZAP, poof, gone! I know high intense UVC light kills this SARS-CoV-2 virus on surfaces. You might want to read the following article: *"Does UV light kill the new coronavirus?"* By Donavyn Coffey livescience.com. I gleaned from this article, that not all lights are quality controlled. UV lights can be detrimental to your health.

Our new, "normal," means the cats are no longer as excited to see me. They are likely wondering when and if I will ever leave, so they can do whatever mischievous cats do when their Mama is away. But my little one, Mika says, and I am speaking for her, "Mama if you just stay home with me, you'll be okay." She is such a sweetie cuddle-bug. I've said the Mika, "Mama" message so many times while holding her she acts as if the words are intended for, "her" instead of me. Mika desperately wants to explore the great outdoors! I am nervous about red tailed hawks, eagles, owls, cougar, and coyotes. I tell her I cannot risk her getting lost or eaten. That would just devastate me! Her big sis, Chessie,* is a tuxedo with a white stripe down her back. She is, I believe, thought to be a skunk by any predators. She is wise and has outdoors smarts. My little one, on the other hand, not so much, when she's gotten out her ears turn off, and she runs to explore the woods. With everything happening in the world, I don't want to risk being the one responsible for her getting outside and possibly lost or eaten by a predator. It would take a great deal of therapy, and even then...I just don't want to think about that happening.

My cat Tiger was lifted by an owl right in front of me one evening. I screamed bloody murder and the owl dropped him. I will never ever forget that night. Tiger lived for 20 years. 1976-1996. He traveled with us wherever my dad was stationed. My dad served in the Air Force, retiring Chief Master Sergeant. Tiger's life was full of adventure having lived in Illinois, Texas, Japan, California, and lastly here in Washington State. When Tiger died (my first baby) it was just before my firstborn son was born. He was an awesome cat! I miss him so, so much, along with all the other pets we've lost through the years- My white copper eyed Persian cat Todo, aka Yuki Boku, 15 years and hamsters Zhu-Zhu, Zupster, Zumiez, and Zak- Each living their estimated 2-3 life expectancy.

*(I was reviewing this book, making little changes here and there when a large hawk had the gall to land on our stoop. I am going to keep Chessie inside too! I asked Dave if he would build a cat fortress so they both can be safe. He added it to the, "Honey-do" list.)

Wishing I could just visit with my friends again. Hug like we used to, go out to lunch, have tea parties, and celebrate birthdays together. I have been baking separate Birthday cakes for my immediate family to blow out their candle wishes. Actually, come to think of it, blowing out candles on a separately made personal cake makes good sense. Perhaps we should have been celebrating Birthdays this way all along!

My family is planning on having a BIG Birthday Bash for everyone once things simmer down with Covid-19. I am so very much looking forward to that day!

Washing hands, my little version:  Happy Birthday to me, Covid19 NOT me, Happy Birthday, Happy Birthday, Happy Birthday to me! And many moorre! Drum roll...

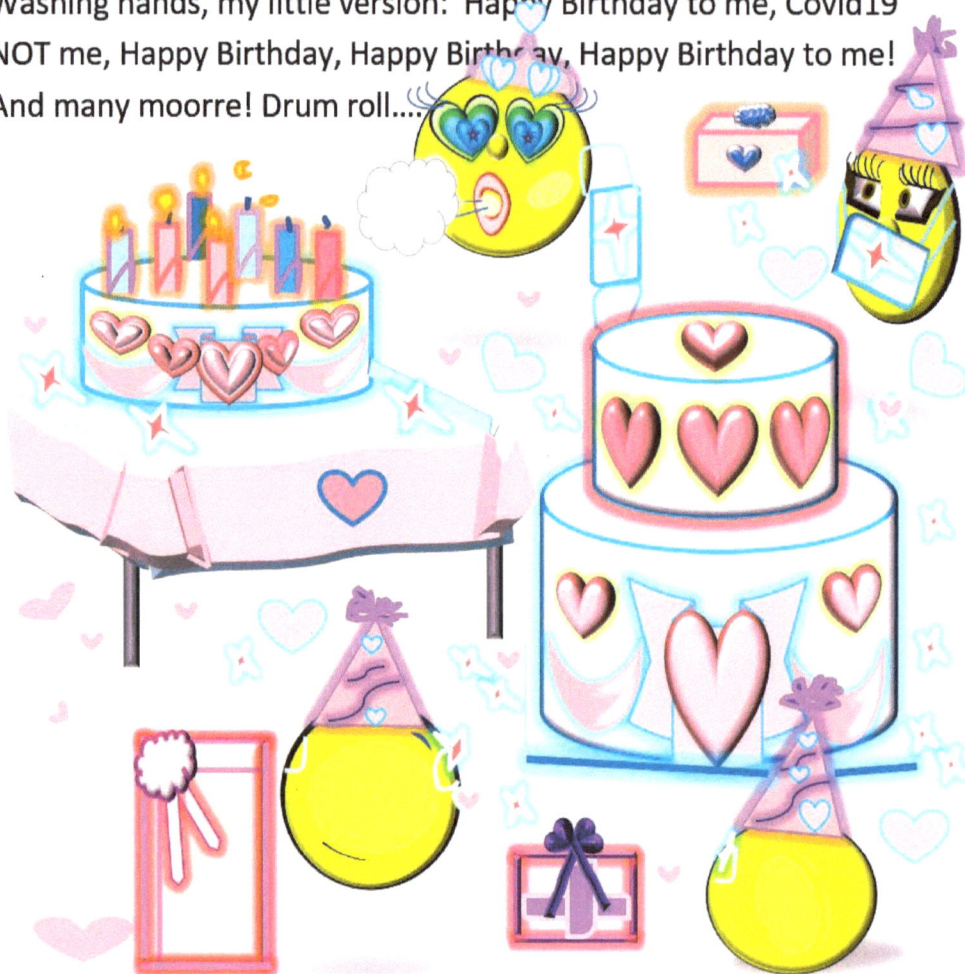

## Flattening the Curve...

It is relatively easy, stay home as much as possible. Socially, this really sucks! We have our phones, Zoom, FaceTime, Netflix, for entertainment- The sanctity of homes (hopefully) no matter how humble, to take care of and **sterilize** regularly, (oh, the joy of house-work!) We have crafts, unfinished projects, books we never had time to read, getting ourselves creative musically, (my heart hasn't been into it.) or other forms of art, or possibly learning a new language. My husband has made three picnic benches, painted a shed and re-sided and painted a small barn, he also put in a new pet door for the cats. I said I managed to do 4 hanging baskets, but actually I also did 3 for my mom for Mother's Day. It was a struggle, as I was feeling really down with everything going on. Some of my pony packs dried up, and I had to purchase more plants for the delay in my planting.

I know it isn't, "normal" to be kept apart from those you love-Especially our parents. I can count on one hand the amount of times I've seen my parents. The last time I put a big blanket between us I hugged my mom and then hugged my dad. He has COPD, a smoker for as long as I've been alive, and longer. For two weeks solid, I wor-ried whether or not I had given him the virus asymptomatically. I felt selfish, and foolish for breaking my own strict rules when it came to protecting my parents. My dad has expressed how he doesn't want anyone to feel responsible or guilty if he were to become infected. This is a "new normal" and it is taking a major adjustment for all of us. (Yes, even for those introverts out there.) So we stay home more often than not, what else? When we are out in public it is important to wear a mask. (Not funny ha, ha Halloween masks) A breathable cotton mask (preferably made with quilters cotton) and if possible, containing a pocket for disposable PM2.5 filters. Masks should be washed daily or alternated. It is better to make or purchase masks where it is obvious which side is intended for the inside. In other words, the mask shouldn't be made from just one pattern of fabric. Get creative. I have a stack of brand new, "granny panties" my husband picked up for me that sadly don't fit. Ugh! –Masks? -Why not.

💗 If everyone is doing their part, **no exceptions,** thecurve will indeed flatten. ——————————————→

Wash your hands frequently, or have hand sanitizer readily available; avoid touching your face, picking your nose; blow your nose into a tissue, and throw away immediately or flush; Cough and sneeze into the crook of your arm (If at all possible); one might even consider wearing eye protection, glasses instead of contacts or aface shield. A thermometer and a fingertip pulse oximeter are also helpful to have on hand. Covid-19 can be transmitted through the eyes. I have read this and heard it many times. Since I wear contacts I have really paid attention to the detail of eye transmission. However, I'm not seeing many people shielding their eyes in public. The following is just one of many sources. aao.org stands for American Academy of Ophthalmology.

"Eye Care During the Coronavirus Pandemic COVID-19 American Academy of Ophthalmology" May 22, 2020 aao.org

If you're on the Frontline, you likely know to wash your clothes/uniform when you get home and shower ASAP; leave your work shoes on the porch. Being ever alert that the pandemic is the real deal even if you personally haven't been affected by it is the way to live this, "new normal." Don't let your guard down. Gently remind your loved ones when they have a lapse in judgement. And have them be mindful to do the same for you. We are creatures of habit. Remember, "Fist bumps!" Go easy on yourself. Try to find something to smile about. Count your blessings. It may helpful to journal, talk to friends on the phone regularly. Consider your passions. If you are unemployed, of no choice of your own, think about taking online classes. Who knows, it might even lead to a new and even better career than what you've been put on the sidelines for.

This is a time to reflect, and find purpose. Seek out others who share your interests. Journal, write down your hopes and dreams. Connect with those you care about. If you haven't heard from a friend or loved one in a long while reach out, give them a call. My mom can always tell when something is the matter with me. When I am feeling slumped, ill, or depressed, I tend to hunker down and shut the world out. It isn't healthy of course, but it is natural for us to withdraw when feeling out of sorts. Seven months of this has got many of us feeling out of sorts.

It might do each of us some good to, "unplug" from the internet, turn off the TV, and find solitude and escape in a good book or take a walk in nature. It is important when venturing outside, to bring your mask, as you never know who might cross your path without protection. You'll want to be on alert. Your efforts to, "flatten the curve" serve as good examples for those still needing a little nudge to show that they, too, really care.


**Do I have SARS-CoV-2, novel coronavirus?**

You may not ever know whether or not you've been infected with SARS-CoV-2, novel coronavirus - Just as I am still unsure of whether or not I had it. You can be completely symptomless, and still have novel coronavirus. It bears repeating, a **completely symptomless, asymptomatic person** can still **spread** the novel coronavirus**!** Hence the **importance of wearing masks**. On the upside most people who become infected generally have mild cases. However, there have been perfectly fit, athletic types who've been knocked for a loop with this virus. This virus isn't something to take lightly, or assume people are overreacting to, some say the virus if overhyped, or not nearly as bad as people make it out to be. It is BAD! It can take you out, or it can spare you and leave you with bizarre on-going symptoms: Tiredness, shortness of breath, and feelings of not being your regular self. Those with lingering effects are known *as long haulers*. We should all act as if we have Covid-19 with our preventative actions and interactions.

Please check out your state's **Department of Health** for detailed information about Covid-19 and symptoms/expectations. If feeling depressed or suicidal please reach out to a friend or your physician. (National Suicide Hotline 1-800-273-8255), Available 24 hours, both English and Spanish assistance.

**For those still balking at the notion of required masks in public...** Please read the following article:

*"Can You Be Medically Exempt from Wearing a Face Mask? Health Experts Weigh In" PS: Those ADA "Face Mask Exemption Cards"? Totally Fake. By: Claire Gillespie, health.com*

Within this article, the CDC directs, "cloth face coverings should not be placed on young children under age 2, anyone who has trouble breathing, or is unable to remove the mask without assistance." The caveat to this is if a person truly cannot wear a mask, for whatever health reason claimed, or has trouble breathing, they likely are too fragile to be in public space in the first place. In other words, Covid-19 could be the death of them. "Staying home to stay healthy" is their best defense and ours too, by the way.

I am really feeling the angst this pandemic is having on our daily lives. It would appear we've taken certain freedoms for granted. I have had to tell myself calmly to, "just breathe." Having something covering our mouths and noses is an adjustment we really just have to make for our own protection and the protection of others. If you are finding your mask difficult to breathe through try a different mask. There are many different masks on the market now. Some are very well made and are comfortable to wear. This is a difficult time for all of us in one degree or another. I empathize with young parents right now who are trying to jostle work and take care of their infants and children. Mine are young adults. They are essentially out of my hands. I still worry about them though.

I take Covid-19 very seriously, and you should too! I can almost hear my husband saying, "Honey, I think they get it now." I sure love that man. I hope we both can survive this to have many more years together. We've been married for over 30 years! Two hearts as 💗

I wasn't able to get vaccinated when Swine Flu reared its ugly head in 2009. There was a limited supply reserved for pregnant women, and the elderly, due to vaccine shortages. A young vivacious girl, no more than five years old, was visiting at my parent's house with her mom and little sister, she became ill with the Swine Flu, and that was that, she died. I'm not certain if I became infected from her or not. I just know it nearly killed me too. I had severe pneumonia, complete incontinence, and felt as if my body had been pummeled. I reached out to a friend who was a nurse, she told me I better get to the doctor, as this was serious, and people were dying. I went to the doctor, he swabbed me, checked me over, and then told me with his back toward me, I had Swine flu. He sent me home with nothing but a diagnosis. I called my friend to tell her and she said to request another doctor. So I did. It took all the energy I had just to go in the first time, but I was driven back down again. On the second visit I was prescribed a Combivent inhaler, and a very strong cough expectorant. I think it important that you know I don't smoke. My lungs should have been healthy, and yet… I became deathly ill. And this is with a virus that had/has a vaccine – A Swine Flu vaccine in very short supply.

NOTE: A vaccine for SARS-CoV-2 novel coronavirus, which can lead to Covid-19, a respiratory disease, on the other hand, is still in the works, and being tested. In other words, in the meantime we are at the mercy of this %*&# virus!


**On YouTube.com:** Reputable and reliable Science based sources for the Coronavirus Covid-19 to keep you up to date and informed are listed below:

Dr. Anthony Fauci          Dr. Roger Seheult, MedCram
Dr. John Campbell          Dr. Sanjay Gupta

**School is in Session; BUT WHERE?**

Summer will soon turn into fall. There is a huge debate as to whether or not parents should send their kids back to school. I was able to find an article about this very topic on the CDC site. If you have school-aged children, I want to encourage you to read the CDC's take on it. *"Schools & Child Care Plan, Prepare, and Respond"* <u>Statement on the importance of Reopening America's Schools this Fall.</u> For what it is worth, here is my take on it - Seeing as the spread of this novel coronavirus is running rampant; I think a rush to get the kids back in school would be a, "HUGE" mistake! -I am remembering the young 5-year old that died from Swine flu in 2009, she was a happy go lucky little girl. Her young life snuffed out! Just like that. I believe the most recent Covid-19 death of a nine-year old Florida girl, thought to be the state's youngest, should be taken into consideration. In addition, California just announced their first Covid-19 teen death. The notion of kids going back to school…patience is a virtue people…

## WE HAVEN'T GOT A VACCINE YET!!!

Why put the, "cart before the horse?" Our children are feeling just as out of sorts as we are, but is it really worth the risk of them getting the virus and bringing it home? I don't think so! Online learning-is going to be crucial until we can ALL be vaccinated. I am also thinking about how defiant kids can be. I can just see a disgruntled, "misbehaving child" removing his or her mask and begin coughing, or spitting at their perceived enemy. It is incredulous that there are people in authority, "sugarcoating" the issue at hand. These are tough times, but we really need to use common sense. We've seen grown adults acting out doing the very same things. It is appalling. We are going to have to knuckle down, and take care of those we love. They grow up fast enough as it is! Mine are 18 and 23.

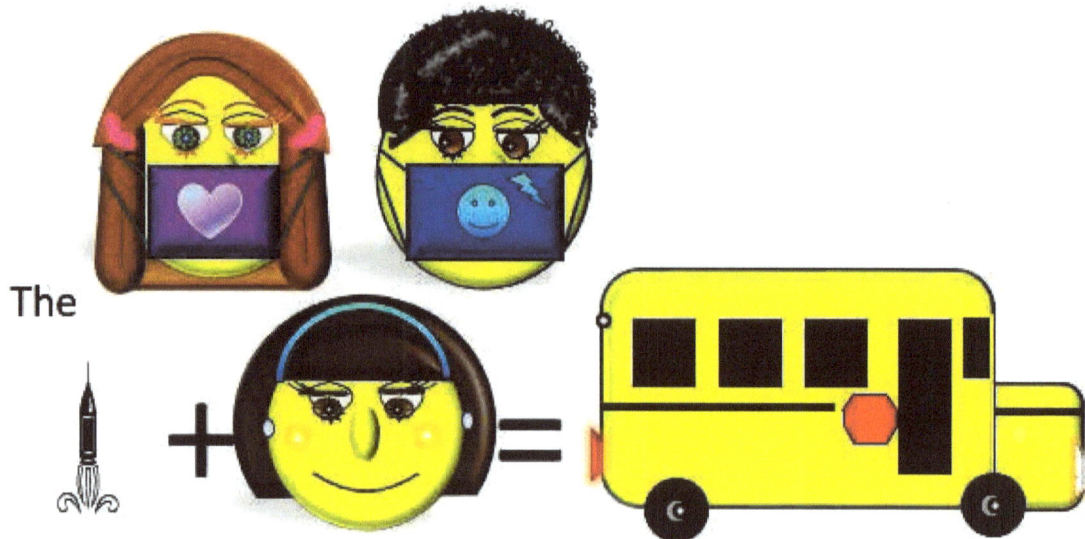

The

NO VACCINE 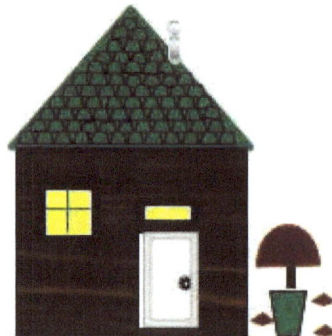 =

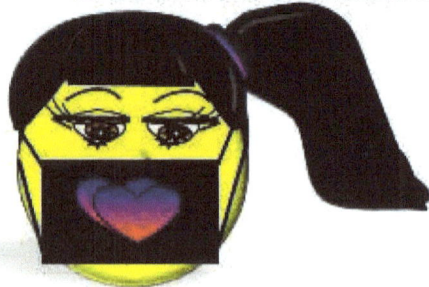

= Home School

= Online Classes

= Distance Learning

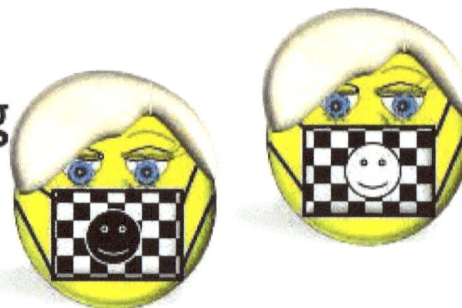

**In Conclusion:**

It is truly humbling, and eye opening, to see the impact the Pandemic, is having on ALL of our lives here in the United States and ALL around the world. It is not only affecting us physically, but also mentally, and emotionally- It can be very draining. I read the news, and am beside myself that there are still those out there determined to party and hoo-haw! - While many of us are doing our best to be responsible in our actions and deeds. I have read that likely upwards of 80% of the world's population will get the coronavirus Covid-19, before a safe and reliable vaccine is available. That leaves only 20% coming through this pandemic unscathed. These percentages are not written in stone. To reiterate, from earlier, we have the POWER to protect ourselves and our loved ones. We **can** and **must together** prevent the spread of this deadly novel coronavirus.

There are several volunteers who have stepped up to be the, "guinea pigs," in the pursuit of a vaccine that will work. I would say more like stepped up to be America's Super Heroes!

**Breaking news:** Final test of Moderna's coronavirus vaccine—in 30,000 volunteers-- gets underway July 27, 2020, *LA Times*

💗We are in this together, each and every one of us.💗

💗**Humankind** - "Human" and "kind" two descriptive words that should naturally go together. With compassion, patience, and determination, respect, and love…. Human + Kind = Human Race, Humanity

Please, America, let's keep our chin up and keep the faith; we know that this too shall pass. We are ALL in this together, and together we will get through this pandemic! If we set our minds to it, we can achieve it. There are plenty of talented brainy people working around the clock to come up with a viable effective vaccine. The total Vaccines in Development now is "157" per ncov2019live.com up by two since the start of this VisualPerspective Exercise and shared journey. People are starting to take this novel coronavirus seriously.

I hope that you have found the exercises to be helpful from a VisualPerspective. (two words needing space like us) ☺ I personally found the exercises to be very revealing of the impact Covid-19 is having here in the USA, especially from the "home county" VisualPerspective. I imagined the people passing me by in the city- gone, deceased, dead, finito! And not just in my city- the whole County! Please share your map with someone still in denial. If you decided to continue tracking you are getting a perspective that has been brought home and condensed into one state, your state specifically.

I believe in the power of prayer. I believe in a Higher Power commonly referred to as GOD. I believe in the power of unity. **Unity** as defined by the *Oxford American Dictionary* is the state of being united or joined as a whole. The United States of America, united in the fight against Covid-19. Too many lives have been lost. All of our lives have been impacted. There is so much grief, and grieving. There are far too many left as widows and widowers, children who have lost a parent(s) or grandparents...it goes on and on...it is time to say, ENOUGH ALREADY!!!

**Breaking News:** "Today, July 29, 2020 *National Geographic* Exclusive: Buddy, first dog to test positive for Covid-19 in the US has died."

Man's best friend. Buddy is one dog of how many more?

It saddens me beyond belief that so many people have lost their lives to Covid-19, and continue to do so, even as I type these words. Now is the time, America, to truly form a unified nation, with a MISSION. A MISSION to do everything in our power to, "Stay home, to stay healthy." Limit our comings and goings to the bare ass minimum. Give one another the space needed to flatten the curve, be helpful to neighbors in need. Do you have an elderly neighbor who perhaps is too shy to ask for your help? You needn't wait for them to ask you; offer to buy groceries, offer to help with yard maintenance, perhaps your elderly neighbor just needs someone to talk to? There are so many people suffering right now. The grief is and can be near unbearable. Compassion, in this time of crisis, is paramount. We cannot avoid the truth of the matter. And the truth of the matter is **we need one another**.

With Conviction and Heartfelt Determination, Shalom

Cheri Lemley

Washington State

P.S. It is my prayerful hope to God that you won't have to trace too many counties in your State in relation to the United States as a whole. We are in a Battle for our Lives! Let's not only try to survive this year,

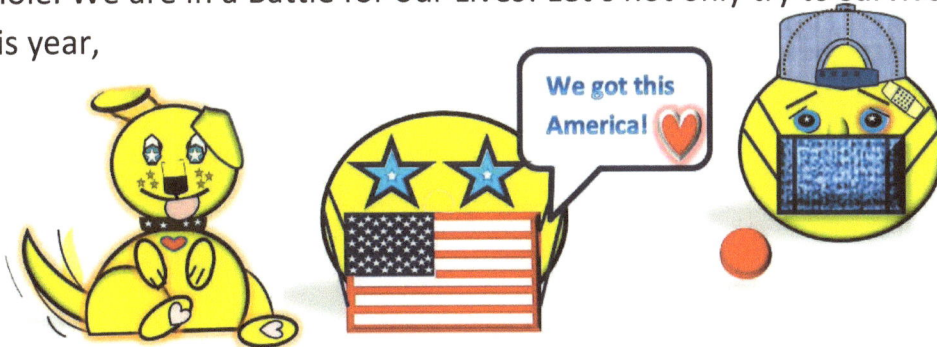

But thrive, by <u>avoiding</u> the virus altogether!

## Please, Will You Wear a Mask?

It's an easy task.

You need not ask me twice.

I'll wear my mask

In the public space

My mask may save my life.

My mask may save your life;

And his, and hers

Both young and old

My mask may save their lives.

So because I care

I'll wear my mask

For me, for you, for them

For the health of us here in the USA

And those around the World,

I'll wear my mask for All and

Say, Thank You, Yes, Thank You!

When you wear your mask

And I wear mine,

And others do the same,

We're ALL together saving LIVES

And that's a beautiful thing!    - Cheri Lemley 💗

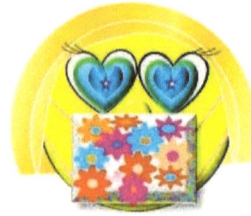

Behind This Mask

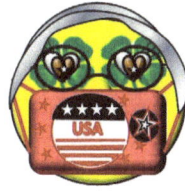

Behind this mask is a person
She wants to live
She has so much more
She wants to give!
So much living
Yet unlived!

Behind this mask is a person
He wants to live
He has so much more
He wants to give!
So much living
Yet unlived!

Behind this mask
I am smiling
My eyes they tell you so.
I see you too,
Are smiling, your eyes they tell me so.

Your eyes tell me you
Want to live!
You, too have so much more
You want to give!
So much living
Yet unlived!

We are wearing
Our masks
Not because it is Mandatory
We are wearing our masks by Choice.
We want to LIVE! –Cheri Lemley

## Lives Matter – My Thoughts in Free Verse

It should go without saying that Black Lives matter.

It should go without saying that Blue Lives matter, aka police officers.

It should go without saying that All Lives matter. It should go

without saying and yet...

We are at a crossroads.

A worldwide pandemic without rhyme or reason Covid-19 is

either benign or deadly

—The value of human life? Spreads asymptomatically, with or without symptoms

Protesters are either peaceful or destructive/deadly

—The value of human life? Spreads by words and actions

Police either uphold the law with compassion or with no regard/deadly

—The value of human life? Spreads by core values and moral fiber

We are our own worst enemy, when we hurt others with a disregard for human life

— our actions or lack of actions (no masks, or social distancing)
— via our words and actions, (destructive protests)
— lack of core values and moral fiber (morally and ethically bankrupt police officers)-prejudiced, and biased

A vicious cycle unbroken. History repeating itself again, and again...

We should be wise to the ugliness no matter where it stems.

Love should prevail. People should be held accountable.

And yet.... Some will insist the battle is, "Good against evil." Who? Whom?

A person may not believe as you do, and or have the same political viewpoints. They are human, just as you are human. Lives should be valued and viewpoints respected.

We have a right to, "freedom of speech" but we should each and every one of us consider the impact of our words spoken. And be a good example to others.

There is a Golden Rule we should all adhere to—

"Treat Others the Way You Want to Be Treated."

For as long as there is division, for as long as there is name calling and a "holier than thou" attitude, we will all stay on this destructive path to nowhere, to never having true peace, and harmony. People are people. Imperfect and falling short of the mark, as some would put it. Hot, Lukewarm or cold, as others would put it.

Believer or unbeliever...

"Live and let live." Forgive, and heal. Respect one another. Appreciate the efforts of the Peace Makers. Listen and learn. There are grains of truth in every perspective—life's experiences do determine our beliefs and actions. We should stop and ask ourselves

Am I helping or hurting the situation at hand?

How can I make a difference without causing my brother or sister undue pain, distress, or loss of life?

What more can I do to show respect and value for human life?

It starts by looking in the mirror. It starts by taking stock of who we are and what kind of person we want to be. It starts with the man, woman, or child's reflection looking back from the mirror.

Lives matter. My life matters, as does Yours, His and Hers or however One Identifies. –Cheri Lemley

# How to Make a Face Mask

What you will need:

Cotton fabric – good quality (preferably

quilting cotton) Rope elastic, beading cord

elastic, 1/8" flat elastic

Cut elastic 7" long and tie a knot at each end (if you are using flat elastic, do not knot the ends.)


You can make 2 sizes: Adult or child


1. Cut 2 pieces – 9x6 for adult or 7.5x 5 for child and put right sides of cotton fabric together.
2. Starting at the center of the bottom edge, sew to the first corner and stop. Sew the elastic with the edge out into the corner. A few stitches forward and back will hold this.
3. Sew to the next corner and stop. Bring the other end of the same elastic to the corner and sew a few stitches forward and back.
4. Now sew across that top of the mask to the next corner. Again, put in elastic with the edge out.
5. Sew to the next corner and sew in the other end of the same elastic.
6. Sew across the bottom leaving about 1.5" to 2" open. Stop, cut the thread. Turn inside out.
7. Pin 3 tucks on each side of the mask – making sure tucks are in the same direction.
8. Sew around the edge of the mask twice.
   This pattern was given to me from Philomena Lund, who found it in the *Sequim Gazette*.
   You can find more patterns at **threadsmonthly.com**, Sara Maker

# WORKSHEETS

_____

_____

_____

_____

_____

_____

_____

_____

_____

_____

_____

_____

_____

_____

_____

_____

_____

# MY 2020-21 PANDEMIC EXPERIENCE

_____

_____

_____

_____

_____

_____

_____

_____

_____

_____

_____

_____

_____

_____

_____

_____

_____

_____

# Acknowledgements

Thank You, Avi Schiffmann for providing the Coronavirus Dashboard **ncov2019.live.** Your site provides vital information on the statistics of Covid-19 here and around the world. Your site also provided the inspiration to create my VisualPerspective exercises.

Please, "Buy Avi a cup of Coffee." 💜

My husband David, "Held down the fort" provided me the time and space to continue working on this book, night and day sometimes even into the wee hours. My tea warm-ups and little plates of fruit and snacks were the sustenance needed to keep forging ahead. Shoulder rubs and kisses also helped in my tired yet resolved determination to see this book through to completion. Thanks Honey for your support. 💜

I am thankful to have Martha McKeeth Ireland, my long time neighbor and friend, for agreeing to edit my book, and assist with the publishing aspect of it. I am also grateful for Martha's willingness to tackle the VisualPerspective exercises. By doing so her input helped me to realize the Map information needed to be in blue. Thank You Martha for all your help and support. *Behind This Mask* poem was inspired by our, as you called it, "Mask to Mask" editing sessions. *Martha has books available on Amazon. 💜

I also want to acknowledge my son's girlfriend Kayla Dudley for her willingness to attempt to do the exercise(s). Kayla became overcome with emotion when she inadvertently wrote down the World's deceased number instead of the United States. (Both the World and United States statistics are devastating!) Her inadvertent error however, brought to light that others might do the same; I rewrote the **ncov2019.live** instructions to be very specific and detailed. Kayla also made me aware that not everyone will be able to handle seeing the VisualPerspective maps. I get that. For me personally, it was very impactful. The news has been grim. People are still acting recklessly. I felt an overwhelming urgency to get the exercises on paper as I strongly felt it would be beneficial to the public. 💜

Marife, the "Mission" is complete. The social distanced Birthday lunch we had planned though delayed and very belated has not been forgotten - The Pantry, for Thai pizza and delicious salads. I haven't seen my dear friend in months. I am cautiously optimistic that we can order to go, keep our distance, and enjoy a little bit of normalcy. 💜

Marilynn Evans, thank you for your willingness to create the book cover for this important topic of Covid-19. You are an amazing digital artist, and I am humbled and ever grateful to have you on board. To try and format the book cover myself...let's just say it is way out of my comfort zone. I am also relieved, beyond words, that your skills include the ability to convert the color of my illustrations from RGB to the print-able color palette of CYMK. The "computer gremlins" met their match. With deep gratitude for your going above and beyond the original request for help. I love your waving cat! Thank you for allowing me to use your version of my original. Also thanks for your willingness to add the Worksheet pages and My 2020-21 Pandemic Experience pages. With Much Love and Appreciation, Cheri. 💜

## To the Reader,

I hope you have found the exercises helpful. If you and I manage to sway even one disbelieving person with the VisualPerspective exercises we will have accomplished the MISSION! Please share your map with someone in doubt. Together we can educate others about the Covid-19 pandemic. It only takes one person infected with the virus to become a "Super spreader." One infected person could soon become seven, and the most vulnerable among us the elderly and those with underlying medical conditions, would be most at risk of having severe complications and even death from Covid-19. Asymptomatic spread of the novel coronavirus is what makes the infectious virus especially problematic. You don't know who may have it, you yourself, or the others you come in contact with. The thought of being responsible for another person's demise makes me shudder. Let's just act like we have it, and keep it to ourselves. And if you do actually have Covid-19, I hope you have a swift recovery.
In My Prayers, Cheri Lemley 💜

# Biographies

**Cheri Lemley** is the wife of David Lemley and the mother of two sons, David and Robert. She writes poetry and short stories none of which have been published, as yet. Cheri is a pianist and currently has two complete music books sitting on the back burner while this more pressing topic of Covid-19 is addressed. Those music books, both forthcoming, are titled, "A Day at the Carnival" Books I and II each containing 12 original piano pieces. Cheri has a love for the arts. She, as mentioned in this book, created the music for *Silent Sky*. She played the character Emily in the Olympic Theatre Arts production of *"Lark Eden"* and was in a local production of *"Joseph and the Technicolor Dreamcoat."* Cheri was involved with two Sequim Readers Theatre plays *"The Last Lifeboat"* first presented on the Olympic Peninsula about the sinking of the Titanic 100 years ago in 2012, and *"A Century of Sequim."* Cheri volunteered at the local radio station KSQM and has two piano pieces used as bed music. *"Tears for Sendai"* is used in the Tsunami emergency preparedness radio production in March; also a piano piece titled, *"Resolve to Overcome"* is bedded into a KSQM production. Cheri was a member of Seattle Children's Hospital Guild, a past member of TOPS, a weight loss group. While in the group Cheri created several songs, poems, and skits for celebrations. Cheri grew up moving from one base to another, as her father served in the Air Force. When Cheri lived on Edwards AFB, CA, she was a Security Guard for NASA and had the honor of guarding the Space Shuttle. She became a caregiver while living in Sequim and has worked as a nanny and an events planner.

**Martha McKeeth Ireland** provides writer services, including editing, proofreading, formatting, design, and assistance with self-publishing; and writes western novels, short stories and articles. She self-published her first western series, *The Trail of the Snake*, in two versions, a two-volume paperback set, and a four-eBook series on Amazon Kindle. Her *Trail* books are action-adventure, murder mystery set in the 1880s. They start along the Snake River in southern Idaho, where she is from originally. She especially enjoys creating in-depth characters and complex plotlines. Her writing career progressed from writing and editing *The Idaho Challenge*, a monthly publication of the Idaho Allied Christian Forces (1967-74); *Service Business*, a Seattle-based quarterly trade journal (1981-88); and the *Peninsula Business Journal* (1989-95). After serving as a Clallam County commissioner 1996-1999, she was a freelance columnist for the *Peninsula Daily News* for more than a dozen years. Martha lives in the Carlsborg area of Clallam County with her husband, horse, cats and cows. She is the mother of two adult children and grandmother of four. She is active in Olympic Peninsula Christian Writers, Peninsula

Evangelical Friends Church, Clallam County Republican Party and Republican Women of Clallam County; and is a member of Sequim Prairie Grange.

**Marilynn Evans,** born and raised in Michigan, currently resides in Sequim, WA. After she and her husband retired from careers in Southern California 20 years ago, they travelled to all 50 states, Canada and Mexico, mostly in their RV, and to Europe, China and Egypt. She has thousands of pictures to prove it! Also hundreds of pictures of flowers from her garden.  What to do with all these photos led to exploring new methods of photography and post digital processing. The computer and the internet have given her the opportunity to try new methods and create her own style. The idea is not to use an artistic approach to cover up bad photography but to enhance it to a WOW factor, using a computer as another venue for "making art." Marilynn says, *"The screen is my canvas, the mouse is my brush. I could paint or take amazing photographs but I choose to combine these two forms of creativity on a computer for timely results."* After studying a photo at length it tells her what it wants to become. The she applies various techniques learned over the years. It is this artistic approach to photography that she follows in her work that may be seen at www.flickr.com/photos/mkevans. Prints and framed originals may be purchased from her or the Blue Whole Gallery in Sequim where her work is being displayed.

# Works Cited

""Scott Fahlman, Inventor Of the Emoticon, Calls Emoji "Ugly' :'-(." 2012. Special Interest.

""Shigetaka Kurita: The man who invented emoji"." 2018. News.

"11 Alive "Rayshard Brooks shooting police bodycam footage from Wendy's parking lot"." 14 June 2020. *YouTube.* Smartphone. June 2020.

Ailee. "Just Look For You." *Sweetest Thing.* By Ailee. 19.

Associated Press. *"Final test of Moderna's coronavirus vaccine gets underway".* News. Las Angeles: Las Angeles Times, July 27, 2020. Smartphone.

Campbell, Dr. John. "Dr. John Campbell." n.d. *YouTube.* Smartphone. 2020.

Carney, Kristen and Morales, Anthony. *www.washington-demographics.com Cubit, demographic data provider.* n.d. Smartphone. July 2020.

CDC. ""Schools & Child Care Plan, Prepare, and Respond"." 24 July 2020. *CDC.* Smartphone.

*CDC.gov.* n.d. Smartphone. 30-31 July 2020.

Charbonneau, Madeline. ""UNPROTECTED 40 Worshippers Infected With COVID-19 After Alabama Revival." 26 July 2020. *Daily Beast.* 2020.

*Chocolate.* Dir. Lee Hyung-min. NetFlix. 2019. South Korean drama.

Coombs, Luke. "Six Feet Apart (Lyric Video)." *https://LC.lnk.to/SFAAY.* By Luke Coombs. 2020. YouTube.

"coronavirus.wa.gov." 2020. Smartphone. 10 Aug 2020.

Fauci, Dr. Anthony. "American Association for Cancer." 21 July 2020. *YouTube.* Smartphone. 31 July 2020.

*For the Beauty of the Earth.* By Folliott S.: Chatterton, William Pierpoint. Perf. Cheri Lemley (prerecorded). OTA, Sequim. Nov 2019. Piano.

Galat, Mathew. "the JaYoe Nation. "Coronavirus Travel Ban| Flying from China to USA"." 2 Feb. 2020. *YouTube.* Smartphone. 2020.

Gearan, Anne, Lati, Marisa, and Dupree, Jacquiline. *"US passes 4 million corona virus cases a pace of new infections roughly doubles.".* News. Washington D.C.: Washington Post, www.washingtonpost.com, 2020. Smartphone.

"Happy Birthday to You-Wikipedia." n.d. *en.m.wikipedia.org.* Facts.

"Indiatimes. "COVID-19: See How Coronavirus Infection Spread When You Sneeze Or Cough."." 8 Apr. 2020. *YouTube.* Smartphone.

Jones, Koreana. "Koreana Jones. "Screaming Chinese Reporter in Wuhan"." 1 Feb 2020. *YouTube.* Smartphone.

*KOIN 6 Gov. Jay Inslee issues 'Stay Home, Stay Healthy' order.* 23 March 2020. Smartphone. 2020.

Mena, Kelly, et al. *Trump wears a mask during visit to wounded service members at Walter Reed.* News. Atlanta: CNN Politics cnn.com Cable News Network, 2020. Smartphone.

Mukamal, Reena, S. Sonal Tuli and Kevin McKinney MD. *aao.org American Academy of Opthalmology "Eye Care During the Coronavirus Pandemic.* 22 May 20. Smartphone. 28 July 2020.

National Geographic. *Today, July 29, 2020 National Geographic Exclusive: Buddy, first dog to test positive for Covid19 in the US has died.* Exclusive news. Washington D.C.: National Geographic, 2020. Smartphone.

"National Suicide Hotline 1-800-273-8255." n.d. 10 Aug 2020.

New York Times. "The New York Times. "How George Floyd Was Killed in Police Custody | Visual Investigations." 1 June 2020. *YouTube.* Smartphone.

"Ninja Nerd Lectures. "COVID-19 Coronavirus: Epidemiology, Pathophysiology| APRIL UPDATE." 20 Apr. 2020. *YouTube.* 2020.

Noah, Trevor. "thedailyshow Trevor Noah. "Breonna Taylor's boyfriend did what anyone might do during a home invasion: used his legal firearm to defend himself.Link in bio." 31 July 2020. *Instagram.* Smartphone. 31 July 2020.

Rivas, Kayla. *"Young patient caught coronavirus at party, spread it to grandfather who died.".* Story sourced from original wfaa.com. New York: Fox News, 23 July 2020. Smartphone.

Ruptly. "Ruptly. "USA: Artists complete large Breonna Taylor mural in Annapolis"." 5 July 2020. *YouTube.* Smartphone. 31 July 2020.

Schiffmann, Avi. *"The High Schooler who became a Covid-19 Watchdog."* Brent Crane. 23 Mar. 2020. Smartphone.

—. *Corona Virus Dashboard www.ncovid.live.com.* Jan 2020. Smartphone. 2020.

Seheult, Dr. Roger. "MedCram - Medical lectures Explained CLEARLY." 2020. *YouTube.* 31 July 2020.

Shammas, Brittany, et al. *"US reports more than 1,000 coronavirus deaths in a day for the first time since early June.* News. Washington D.C.: The Washington Post, washingtonpost.com, 2020. Smartphone.

*Silent Sky.* By Lauren Gunderson. OTA, Sequim. 8-24 Nov 2019. Play.

Tang, Hai. "Ergeng TV "Video Diary" [Wuhans] An Infectected Emergncy Room Nurse Episode 25 [Homecoming}." 1 Apr. 2020. *YouTube.* Smartphone. 2020.

Tapp, Tom. *California Coronavirus Update: First Teen Death From Virus Confirmed in State As Death Toll Passes 9,00.* Home/ business/ L.A. Local. Las Angeles: Deadline, 2020. Smartphone.

*who.int.* 11 Feb 2020. Document. 4 July 2020.

Wikipedia. "WikipediA COVID-19 pandemic in Washington (state)." 21 Jan 2020. *en.m.wikipedia.org.* Smartphone. July 2020.

Winningham, Cathleigh. *9-year-old Florida girl believed to be state's youngest COVID-19 death".* News. Putnam County: ClickOrlando.com, 2020. Smartphone.

*www.doh.wa.gov.* n.d. Smartphone. 31 July 2020.

"www.merriam-webster.com." n.d. Smartphone. 11 Aug. 2020.

*www.whowhatwear.com Is nylon spandex breathable? "The 10 Best (and Worst) Fabrics to Wear During Summer.. .* 3 May 2020. Smartphone. 30 May 2020.

(YouTube "How to Make a Fun Shape School Bus Craft| Craft Tutorial)

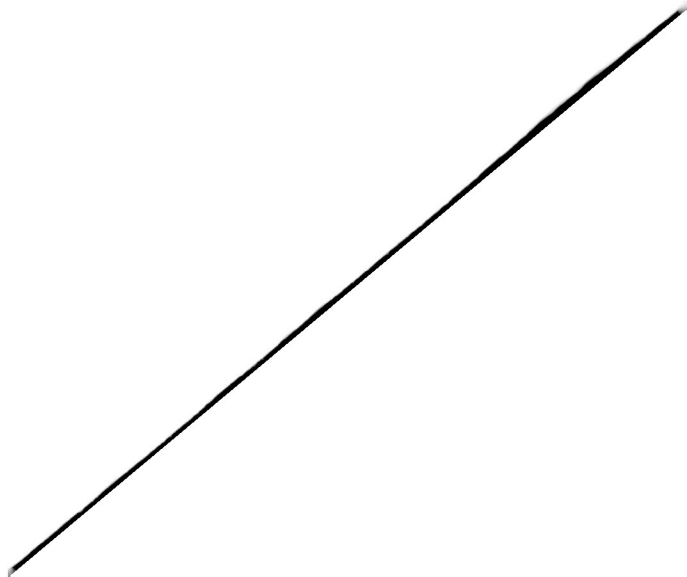

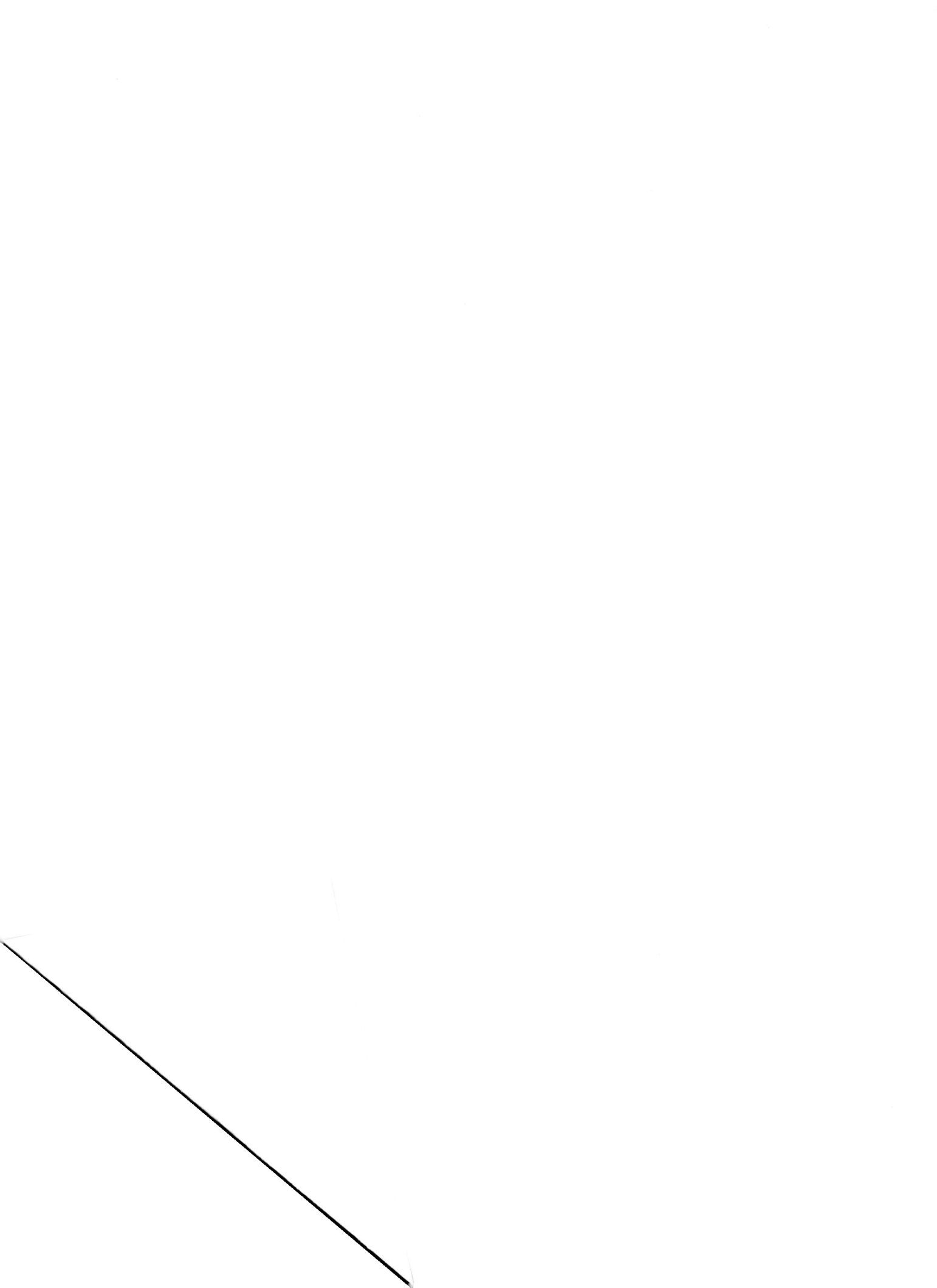